OVERDIAGNOSED

# Overdiagnosed

MAKING PEOPLE SICK IN THE PURSUIT OF HEALTH

### Dr. H. Gilbert Welch
Dr. Lisa M. Schwartz
Dr. Steven Woloshin

BEACON PRESS · BOSTON

Beacon Press
25 Beacon Street
Boston, Massachusetts 02108–2892
www.beacon.org

Beacon Press books
are published under the auspices of
the Unitarian Universalist Association of Congregations.

14 13 12 11     8 7 6 5 4 3 2 1

This book is printed on acid-free paper that meets the uncoated paper ANSI/NISO
specifications for permanence as revised in 1992.

Composition by Wilsted & Taylor Publishing Services

Library of Congress Cataloging-in-Publication Data

Welch, H. Gilbert.
  Overdiagnosed : making people sick in the pursuit of health / H. Gilbert Welch,
  Lisa Schwartz, Steven Woloshin.
     p. ; cm.
  Includes bibliographical references and index.
  ISBN 978-0-8070-2200-9 (hardcover : alk. paper)
  1. Diagnostic errors. 2. Medical misconceptions. 3. Medical screening. I. Schwartz,
Lisa. II. Woloshin, Steven. III. Title.
  [DNLM: 1. Diagnostic Techniques and Procedures—ethics. 2. Early Diagnosis.
  3. Diagnostic Techniques and Procedures—utilization. 4. Early Detection of Cancer—
  ethics. 5. Early Detection of Cancer—utilization. 6. Health Policy. WB 60]
  RC71.3.W45 2011
  616.07′54—dc22                    2010037078

Many names and identifying characteristics of people mentioned in this work have been
changed to protect their identities.

*To my mother,*

*Katharine Smith Welch*

*(1920–2010)*

INTRODUCTION  Our Enthusiasm for Diagnosis    ix

*Chapter 1*    Genesis
*People Become Patients with High Blood Pressure*    1

*Chapter 2*    We Change the Rules
*How Numbers Get Changed to Give You Diabetes,*
*High Cholesterol, and Osteoporosis*    15

*Chapter 3*    We Are Able to See More
*How Scans Give You Gallstones, Damaged Knee Cartilage,*
*Bulging Discs, Abdominal Aortic Aneurysms, and*
*Blood Clots*    32

*Chapter 4*    We Look Harder for Prostate Cancer
*How Screening Made It Clear That Overdiagnosis*
*Exists in Cancer*    45

*Chapter 5*    We Look Harder for Other Cancers    61

*Chapter 6*    We Look Harder for Breast Cancer    73

*Chapter 7*    We Stumble onto Incidentalomas
That Might Be Cancer    90

*Chapter 8*    We Look Harder for Everything Else
*How Screening Gives You (and Your Baby)*
*Another Set of Problems*    102

*Chapter 9*    We Confuse DNA with Disease
*How Genetic Testing Will Give You Almost Anything*    116

*Chapter 10*    Get the Facts    136

*Chapter 11*     Get the System   151

*Chapter 12*     Get the Big Picture   167


CONCLUSION     Pursuing Health with Less Diagnosis   180

ACKNOWLEDGMENTS   192

NOTES   194

INDEX   218

# Our Enthusiasm for Diagnosis

MY FIRST CAR WAS A '65 Ford Fairlane wagon. It was a fairly simple—albeit large—vehicle. I could even do some of the work on it myself. There was a lot of room under the hood and few electronics. The only engine sensors were a temperature gauge and an oil-pressure gauge.

Things are very different with my '99 Volvo. There's no extra room under the hood—and there are lots of electronics. And then there are all those little warning lights sensing so many different aspects of my car's function that they have to be connected to an internal computer to determine what's wrong.

Cars have undoubtedly improved over my lifetime. They are safer, more comfortable, and more reliable. The engineering is better. But I'm not sure these improvements have much to do with all those little warning lights.

Check-engine lights—red flags that indicate something may be wrong with the vehicle—are getting pretty sophisticated. These sensors can identify abnormalities long before the vehicle's performance is affected. They are making early diagnoses.

Maybe your check-engine lights have been very useful. Maybe one of them led you to do something important (like add oil) that prevented a much bigger problem later on.

Or maybe you have had the opposite experience.

Check-engine lights can also create problems. Sometimes they are false alarms (whenever I drive over a big bump, one goes off warning me that something's wrong with my coolant system). Often the lights are in response to a real abnormality, but not one that is especially important (my favorite is the sensor that lights up when it recognizes that another sensor is not sensing). Recently, my mechanic confided to me that many of the lights should probably be ignored.

Maybe you have decided to ignore these sensors yourself. Or maybe you've taken your car in for service and the mechanic has simply reset them and told you to wait and see if they come on again.

Or maybe you have had the unfortunate experience of paying for an unnecessary repair, or a series of unnecessary repairs. And maybe you have been one of the unfortunate few whose cars were worse off for the efforts.

If so, you already have some feel for the problem of overdiagnosis.

I don't know what the net effect of all these lights has been. Maybe they have done more good than harm. Maybe they have done more harm than good. But I do know there's little doubt about their effect on the automotive repair business: they have led to a lot of extra visits to the shop.

And I know that if we doctors look at you hard enough, chances are we'll find out that one of your check-engine lights is on.

### A routine checkup

I probably have a few check-engine lights on myself. I'm a male in my mid-fifties. I have not seen a doctor for a routine checkup since I was a child. I'm not bragging, and I'm not suggesting that this is a path others should follow. But because I have been blessed with excellent health, it's kind of hard to argue that I have missed out on some indispensable service.

Of course, as a doctor, I see doctors every day. Many of them are my friends (or at least they were before they learned about this book). And I can imagine some of the diagnoses I could accumulate if I were a patient in any of their clinics (or in my own, for that matter):

- From time to time my blood pressure runs a little high. This is particularly true when I measure it at work (where blood pressure machines are readily available).
  **Diagnosis: borderline hypertension**
- I'm six foot four and weigh 205 pounds; my body mass index (BMI) is 25. (A "normal" BMI ranges from 20 to 24.9.)
  **Diagnosis: overweight**
- Occasionally, I'll get an intense burning sensation in my midchest after eating or drinking. (Apple juice and apple cider are particularly problematic for me.)
  **Diagnosis: gastroesophageal reflux disease**
- I often wake up once a night and need to go to the bathroom.
  **Diagnosis: benign prostatic hyperplasia**
- I wake up in the morning with stiff joints and it takes me a while to loosen up.
  **Diagnosis: degenerative joint disease**
- My hands get cold. Really cold. It's a big problem when I'm skiing or snowshoeing, but it also happens in the office (just ask my patients). Coffee makes it worse; alcohol makes it better.
  **Diagnosis: Raynaud's disease**

- I have to make lists to remember things I need to do. I often forget people's names—particularly my students'. I have to write down all my PINs and passwords (if anyone needs them, they are on my computer).
**Diagnosis: early cognitive impairment**
- In my house, mugs belong on one shelf, glasses on another. My wife doesn't understand this, so I have to repair the situation whenever she unloads the dishwasher. (My daughter doesn't empty the dishwasher, but that's a different topic.) I have separate containers for my work socks, running socks, and winter socks, all of which must be paired before they are put away. (There are considerably more examples like this that you don't want to know about.)
**Diagnosis: obsessive-compulsive disorder**

Okay. I admit I've taken a little literary license here. I don't think anyone would have given me the psychiatric diagnoses (at least, not anyone outside of my immediate family). But the first few diagnoses are possible to make based solely on a careful interview and some simple measurements (for example, height, weight, and blood pressure).

More are possible if a doctor were to order any one of a number of diagnostic tests for me. Even routine blood work—a complete blood count, an electrolyte panel, and liver function tests—involves more than twenty separate measurements. The chances are good that I would have at least one abnormal value.

And then there's imaging. Lots of people have "abnormal" findings on X-ray studies. If I had a chest X-ray, I wouldn't be surprised if a lung nodule was seen. If I had an abdominal CT scan, I wouldn't be surprised if a cyst on my kidney was found.

Further inspection could reveal more. A colonoscopy might show that I have polyps—as about a third of people my age do. A prostate biopsy might demonstrate a small cancer—which many men have, even if their PSA (prostate-specific antigen) screening tests are normal. And it's a safe bet that my genome contains all sorts of genetic variants.

To be fair, most doctors wouldn't order any imaging studies; some might have skipped the routine blood work. Nonetheless, several of these diagnoses could have been made.

Would I be better off if I were given these diagnoses? I don't think so. Would I be put on prescription medications? Probably. Would I consider this good medical care or bad? I'd say bad. But enough about me. This book is about the millions of Americans who have access to what some would call the best medical care in the world. Of course, there are millions of other Americans whose access is severely limited—the uninsured. This is a real problem, but not the topic of this book. The problems described here are actually less likely to happen to the latter group, simply because they receive less medical care. This book is about the relentless expansion of medicine and our increasing tendency to make diagnoses.

Americans have been trained to be concerned about our health. All sorts of hidden dangers lurk inside of us. The conventional wisdom is that it's always better to know about these dangers so that something can be done. And the earlier we know, the better. That's why we are so enthusiastic about amazing medical technologies that can detect abnormalities even when we think we are well. That's also why we welcome the identification of risk factors, disease awareness campaigns, cancer screening, and genetic testing. Americans love diagnosis, especially early diagnosis.

Not surprisingly, we get more diagnoses today than we did in the past. In fact, we are in the midst of an epidemic of diagnosis. Again, the conventional wisdom tells us that this is good: finding problems early saves lives because we have the opportunity to fix small problems before they become big ones. What's more, we believe there are no downsides to looking for things to be wrong.

But the truth is that early diagnosis is a double-edged sword. While it has the potential to help some, it always has a hidden danger: overdiagnosis—the detection of abnormalities that are not destined to ever bother us.

### Living longer, yet sicker?

Consider the generation of which I am a part—the baby boomers. This is the generation born in the period of increased birthrates that followed World War II. They went on to become leaders in the major social movements of the 1960s—civil rights, feminism, and the Vietnam War protests. They also spawned the counterculture of that era: sex, drugs, and rock and roll. As they aged, they became the dominant culture: they gained political power and amassed large sums of money. Now television ads promise them that they will engage in a new kind of retirement, one in which their dreams won't retire. Just think of the Ameriprise ad featuring the late Dennis Hopper saying, "'Cause I just don't see you playing shuffleboard—know what I mean?" (while the powerhouse organ riff from the classic rock hit "Gimme Some Lovin'" blares in the background). Brings back fond memories of high school. I love it.

But then I saw a piece in the *Washington Post* suggesting that the boomers might indeed need to prepare for a different view of retirement—because they are falling apart.[1] Large national surveys reported that while 57 percent of those born before World War II reported excellent health as they approached retirement, only 50 percent of boomers described themselves in this way. About 56 percent of those born before World War II reported having a chronic condition at retirement; about 63 percent of boomers reported having a chronic condition at the same age. Could boomers be in worse shape than their parents were?

A few weeks later I attended a medical meeting at which one of the participants reported on the Department of Health and Human Services' midcourse review of the program called Healthy People 2010. This is the federal government's effort to increase both the length and the quality of life. Length of life was measured using life expectancy—the average number of years Americans live. Quality of life was measured using healthy life expectancy—the average number of years Americans live free of disease (such as heart disease, stroke, cancer, diabetes, hypertension, and arthritis). The speaker showed a table with data from 1999 to 2002, during which life expectancy had increased by about six months, from 76.8 to 77.2 years. But surprisingly, the healthy life expectancy had *fallen* by a little more than a year, from 48.7 to 47.5.

It looked like the program was getting it only half right: the quantity of life was increasing (people were living longer), but the length of healthy life was decreasing (people were having fewer disease-free years). Could we be living longer, yet be sicker? That is hard to believe. But there is an alternative explanation: we live longer, we are healthier, but we are increasingly more likely to be *told* we are sick.

Some may view diagnosing more people (and treating more people) as the price that has to be paid for most of us to achieve an extension of life. This assumes that early diagnosis and treatment is the only explanation of a longer life span. But because other things are more important (such as not smoking, nutrition, exercise, and medical care for the acutely ill), it's likely that most of this life extension would occur regardless of whether or not there was more diagnosis. And since for many, length of life is not the only goal, questions about whether the health-care system introduces disease and disability into the population become more relevant.

### What this book is about

My mother thinks she knows what this book is about. She is almost ninety and has advanced dementia. A few months ago she picked up my first book and read the title out loud: *"Should I Be Tested for Cancer?"* And then she answered with a resounding *"No!"* (Note: her response is a vast oversimplification of the book's content.)

She asked me what my next book would be about. I attempted to explain it to her. She suggested that it be titled *Should I Be Tested for Anything?* Not that great a title, but it gives you the idea. This book examines the possibility that American medicine now labels too many of us as "sick."

As I've noted, the conventional wisdom is that more diagnosis—particularly, more early diagnosis—means better medical care. The logic goes something like this: more diagnosis means more treatment, and more treatment means better health. This may be true for some. But there is another side to the story. More diagnosis may make healthy people feel more vulnerable—and, ironically, less healthy. In other words, excessive diagnosis can literally make you feel sick. And more diagnosis leads to excessive treatment—treatment for problems that either aren't that bothersome or aren't bothersome at all. Excessive treatment, of course, can really hurt you. Excessive diagnosis may lead to treatment that is worse than the disease.

More specifically, this book is about overdiagnosis. While the term sounds like it means simply "excessive diagnosis," it actually also has a more precise meaning. Overdiagnosis occurs when individuals are diagnosed with conditions that will never cause symptoms or death.

So while I diagnosed myself with a number of conditions a few pages ago, some were not overdiagnoses, since I had symptoms: heartburn, cold hands, and so forth (although they may well constitute excessive diagnoses, given that my symptoms were trivial). But the diagnoses related to slight elevations in blood pressure and weight were not associated with symptoms. They could reflect overdiagnosis. So too could all the diagnoses I might have gotten following subsequent testing. In other words, overdiagnosis can occur only when a doctor makes a diagnosis in a person who has no symptoms referable to the condition. While this can happen when a doctor stumbles onto unexpected diagnoses in the course of an evaluation of unrelated conditions, generally it happens because doctors seek early diagnoses—either as part of an organized screening effort or during routine exams. Thus, overdiagnosis is a consequence of the enthusiasm for early diagnosis.

The trouble is that we doctors don't know if an individual has been overdiagnosed unless that person forgoes treatment, lives the rest of his or her life symptom free, and dies from some other cause. But we do know that if we make more and more diagnoses in a healthy population, we are more likely to overdiagnose.

Overdiagnosis is a relatively new problem in medicine. In the past, people didn't go to the doctor when they were well—they tended to wait until they developed symptoms. Furthermore, doctors didn't encourage the healthy to seek care. The net result was that doctors made fewer diagnoses than they do now.

But the paradigm has changed. Early diagnosis is the goal. People seek care when they are well. Doctors try to detect disease earlier. More people have findings of early disease than of late disease. So we make more diagnoses—including diagnoses in those who have no symptoms. Some of these people are destined to develop symptoms. Others are not—they are overdiagnosed.

So the problem of overdiagnosis stems directly from the expansion of the pool of individuals in whom we make diagnoses: from individuals with disease (those with symptoms) to individuals with abnormalities (those without symptoms). The problem is further aggravated as the definition of what constitutes an abnormality gets increasingly broad.

The objective of this book is to lay out the data on how overdiagnosis occurs, explain why it can be harmful, and explore its root causes. My hope is to help you critically consider the desirability of being turned into a patient prematurely.

Let me be clear about why you should care about overdiagnosis. Since doctors don't know who is overdiagnosed and who is not, overdiagnosed patients tend to get treated. But an overdiagnosed patient cannot benefit from treatment. There's nothing to be fixed—he will neither develop symptoms nor die from his condition—so the treatment is unneeded. An overdiagnosed patient can only be harmed. And the simple truth is that almost all treatments have the potential to do some harm.

### What this book is not about

This book is not about what you should do when you are sick. It is not for the few who are severely ill (those for whom medical care offers a lot), but for the many who are (or used to be) basically well—or those who have one illness and are at risk of being told they have others. Nor is this book an apology for sloppy diagnosis in the sick. Diagnosis is always important when people are suffering, and it's important that it be done well. None of my comments should be construed as suggesting you are better off not being diagnosed when you are sick. Finally, this book is not a condemnation of all of American medicine, nor a call for alternative medicine. I'm conventionally trained in Western medicine, and I believe doctors do a lot of good. If you are sick, you should see one.

### A final note about people and language

Before moving on, I feel obliged to make a few comments about names and words. There are stories in this book: stories about my patients, my friends, and people I've met along the way. The stories are accurate; the names are not. While I have not altered information relevant to the clinical narrative (such as the individual's gender, age, symptoms, and experiences), I have altered information that could potentially identify individuals (such as whether a person is from New York or New Jersey—as my daughter might say, "Like it matters").

Then there is the word *disease*. Although the word has a wide range of interpretations, its origins are quite specific. *Dis-* means "without," and *ease* requires no explanation. A synonym for *disease* might be *discomfort*. Although there are other perfectly legitimate definitions, in this book *disease* will refer to a condition that a person experiences—a sickness, an illness, a disorder that produces symptoms.

The word *abnormality* will serve a distinct purpose. I will use it to describe findings that are considered abnormal in the medical profession yet are not experienced by the individual. Some of the most familiar abnormalities—high blood pressure, high cholesterol—will sometimes be referred to as *conditions* to distinguish them from *diseases*.

Although occasionally I use the broad term *health-care provider*, for simplicity, I tend to use the term doctor. This is not meant to exclude other caregivers. On the contrary, it is important to acknowledge that physician assistants and nurse-practitioners are assuming larger and more important roles in medicine—particularly in the delivery of primary care (where a lot of diagnoses are made).

Finally, some quick notes about pronouns. The most familiar are *he* and *she*. Of course, a patient can be either male or female, as can a doctor (there are now more women than men enrolled at Dartmouth Medical School). I don't know of a satisfactory way to handle the absence of a gender-neutral singular pronoun. *He* or *she* gets pretty awkward after a while; using *they* would upset my mother too much. So when the situation allows (some diseases are gender specific), I alternate between the two.

Then there's *we*. *We* will generally refer to "we doctors" or "we health-care providers." (I'd guess *generally* means "roughly 90 percent of the time" —although I'm not going to bother to calculate it.) I use *we* in an attempt to represent the professional perspective of doctors: what we are taught in medical school, how we are trained as residents, what we learn in practice. In short, I'll try to give you a sense of how we think. Not that we all think alike, but we do all share a common experience, about which you should have some insight.

Occasionally *we* will refer to "we the public." Just like you, I am a member of society and a potential patient. And all of us will face some decision about how we want to interact with medical care. Sometimes I modify the *we* with something like "we the public" when I am attempting to communicate this perspective.

*I* will represent me—the author. But it should be another *we*, as this book is really a collaboration of three authors: Dr. Lisa Schwartz, Dr. Steven Woloshin, and myself. But to avoid the confusion with the other *we*'s requires this sleight of hand. To be clear, our voice encompasses two viewpoints. All three of us are academic physicians: we see patients, we teach students, and we do research. But we are also people, and therefore potential patients. As people, we are concerned about the relentless expansion of the medical profession and the subsequent drive to turn people into patients. It is the melding of these two viewpoints—medical and personal—that provides the motivation for this book.

# CHAPTER 1

# Genesis

*People Become Patients with High Blood Pressure*

MIGHT AS WELL BEGIN AT the beginning. And the beginning of overdiagnosis lies in the diagnosis and treatment of a common condition—hypertension (high blood pressure).

Only one paragraph in and I can already sense the unease in my physician and public health colleagues (*Is he really going to start by suggesting we stop diagnosing hypertension? We're not doing enough to diagnose and treat hypertension now!*). In fact, detecting and treating high blood pressure is one of the most important things we doctors do. And it's true that we don't do enough of it. There are some people with undetected hypertension who would benefit tremendously from treatment.

But it's also true we do too much of it. Some people are diagnosed and treated needlessly—they are overdiagnosed. Hypertension was arguably the first condition for which regular treatment was started in people without symptoms.[1] Prior to the late twentieth century, physicians generally prescribed medicines only to patients with symptoms of disease. But hypertension changed that. Suddenly people with no health complaints—who perceived no health problems—were being given a diagnosis and prescribed treatment. People became patients—it was really a remarkable paradigm shift. Seeking diagnoses of hypertension in those without symptoms provided the opportunity to prevent symptomatic disease in some, but at the cost of making the diagnosis in others who were not destined ever to develop symptoms or die from hypertension. In other words, at the cost of overdiagnosis.

### A condition that warrants treatment

I work at a small Department of Veterans Affairs hospital in White River Junction, Vermont. Earlier in my career, I'd spend one or two months a year taking care of patients who were sick enough to be admitted to the hospital. One evening I admitted a fifty-seven-year-old man who came to the emergency room complaining of severe chest pain. Mr. Lemay told me he had been having increasingly frequent episodes of chest pain; sometimes he had the chest pain when he was walking or otherwise exerting himself, and sometimes he had the chest pain when he was doing nothing at all.

The phrase *chest pain* has almost magical qualities in medicine. It is a powerful catalyst for action; it can trigger a cascade of tests and interventions. That is because chest pain sometimes signals a heart attack—the number-one cause of death in the United States. A patient's mere mention of chest pain impels us to do a number of things very quickly, like provide supplemental oxygen, administer an aspirin, and check an electrocardiogram. Mr. Lemay's electrocardiogram was markedly abnormal. It showed that part of his heart wasn't getting enough oxygen, a sign of an impending heart attack.

But something else was markedly abnormal. His blood pressure was 202/117. Blood pressure is measured using two numbers. The top number (in this case, 202) is called the systolic blood pressure. It reflects the highest pressure in your arteries—the pressure created immediately following the contraction of the heart. The bottom number (in this case, 117) is called the diastolic blood pressure. It reflects the lowest pressure in your arteries—the pressure immediately prior to the contraction of the heart—that is, when your heart is most relaxed. If a doctor is asked, "What is a normal blood pressure?" she'll typically give the numbers 120/80. But doctors see blood pressures higher than this all the time. The question is: At what level is blood pressure abnormal? Most doctors would agree that a systolic pressure over 160 or a diastolic pressure over 90 is abnormally high. And we all would agree that 202/117 is abnormally high. Really high. In fact—really, really high.

Because an impending heart attack was a genuine concern, I admitted Mr. Lemay to the intensive care unit. We gave him medicines to lower his blood pressure, and his chest pain quickly went away. He did not have a heart attack. Well, maybe by today's standards he did. This was in the early 1990s, before we routinely checked troponin levels (a very sensitive indicator of heart damage). Then we made the diagnosis by combining electrocardiogram findings with relatively crude laboratory measurements. My guess is that today we would diagnose Mr. Lemay as having had a small heart attack—a subendocardial myocardial infarction. But all the same, a couple of days later, he went home. That was over fifteen years ago. And he has not been in the hospital since.

Mr. Lemay is now seventy-two. I see him in clinic about twice a year. He's been very healthy. I've done very little for him, except one thing: I've made sure his blood pressure is controlled. It's not glamorous. It's not difficult. It certainly doesn't require a physician (nurses, nurse-practitioners, and physician assistants can do it just as well). But for patients like Mr. Lemay, it's pretty close to being the difference between life and death. While one can never be sure, I am confident that he would have died years ago had his hypertension not been diagnosed and adequately treated. Of course, he came to the emergency room not for the high blood pressure but for the chest pain it caused. But even if he had had no symptoms, simply a sustained blood pressure of 202/117, I would say that treatment saved his life. Let me tell you why I can confidently say that.

### Discovering the effects of hypertension

Although physicians have been able to measure blood pressure for well over a hundred years, they were slow to recognize the dangers of hypertension. President Franklin D. Roosevelt, for example, was known to have high blood pressure—it was recorded as being higher than 200/100 at the time of his re-election in November of 1944—but it is unclear whether his doctors recognized it was a problem. Six months later he developed a hypertensive crisis: a severe headache followed by a loss of consciousness and a measured blood pressure of 300/190. He died shortly thereafter of a massive hemorrhage in his brain.[2]

As late as the 1950s, some expert physicians considered high blood pressure to be essential for some patients: essential to deliver enough blood to vital organs. Insurance companies, however, did recognize the dangers of hypertension at the time—they observed that people with high blood pressure were more likely to die, and they often refused to sell them life insurance policies.[3]

In the mid-1960s, the Veterans Administration (now the Department of Veterans Affairs) decided to study the value of treating people who had hypertension but no symptoms of it. It initiated a VA cooperative study; *cooperative* because these studies involve veterans from multiple VA hospitals. This study identified men (almost all veterans at the time were male) who had been found to have high blood pressure when they were hospitalized for other reasons. The investigators tracked the men's blood pressure after they left the hospital and recruited those whose average outpatient diastolic blood pressure—the bottom number—ranged from 115 to 129 (that is, those who had what we would now call severe diastolic hypertension). Because the idea of giving people medicine for a condition that produced no symptoms was so unusual, the investigators decided to make sure that study participants would actually take the medicine prescribed for them. So before any patient could be enrolled in the study, he had to pass a test to demonstrate that he would take a medicine regularly even if he felt well.

Here's what the test involved. Each prospective participant was given two containers of pills (two because the investigators correctly anticipated that treated patients would require two drugs) along with instructions of how to take each. One pill was an inert sugar pill; the other was vitamin $B_2$ — also known as riboflavin. Two weeks later, the participants met with study personnel, and they counted the pills left in each container. If the correct number remained, the investigators presumed that the medicine had been taken correctly. But they had a second way to check whether prospective participants had taken their medicine: a simple urine examination. Riboflavin imparts a bright yellow color to urine that fluoresces brilliantly under UV light. Nearly half of the prospective participants failed the test and so were not enrolled in the study, as they could not be relied upon to take their medications regularly.

This finding highlights how much of a paradigm shift this was. At that time, people simply didn't take medicines in the absence of symptoms. Now it is the norm. In contemporary studies of hypertension therapy, typically less than 20 percent fail a test of medication adherence.[4]

This VA study was a true experiment: The enrolled participants were divided into two groups, and the group to which each subject was assigned was determined purely by chance. One group received treatment for hypertension (the drug hydrochlorothiazide combined with either reserpine or hydralazine); the other group received placebos (inert sugar pills). The VA cooperative study of the treatment of severe hypertension is considered one of our classic randomized trials. Because discussions of randomized trials will appear throughout this book, figure 1.1 illustrates their basic design. Randomized trials are studies in which enrolled patients are assigned to either receive treatment or not simply by chance. We typically describe this allocation process as being like the flip of a coin; operationally, however, it is accomplished by computer. The word *randomized* is used because the group an individual is assigned to is randomly chosen.

The randomized trial was developed in the 1940s by British epidemiologists, who used it to demonstrate that pertussis vaccine prevented whooping cough and that a drug called streptomycin cured tuberculosis.[5] Unfortunately, the concept was slow to catch on, and we still don't do enough of them. Why do I say this? Because randomized trials are the most reliable way to determine what works in medicine.[6] If members of two groups are similar to each other in every way except one—whether or not they get treatment—

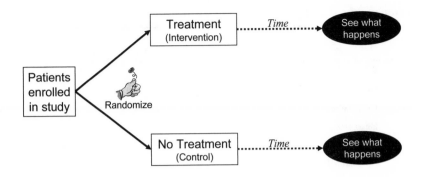

FIGURE 1.1 *Basic Design of a Randomized Trial*

then any differences observed at the end of the trial must be the result of the treatment.

For over two decades we were misled by observations that postmenopausal women who took hormone replacement therapy did better (in terms of just about everything) than those who did not. But when women were finally allocated to hormone replacement therapy or placebo in a randomized trial, we learned the therapy caused more problems than it solved.[7] It is tempting to compare people who take a particular medicine with those who do not, but these groups differ in many important ways other than the fact of treatment. In particular, people who take medicine (that is, those that have access to doctors, can afford the prescription, and choose to take it) tend to be better educated, wealthier, and more attentive to health in general (for example, they exercise more; they smoke less). So while this kind of comparison is easy, it is not fair. People who take preventive medicines are bound to do better than those who don't simply because they are healthier to start with—even if the medicine doesn't help one bit. To avoid this problem, we need to do true experiments: randomized trials.

### The VA randomized trial of treatment for severe hypertension

The VA trial was pretty small by current standards: there were only about 140 enrolled participants. About 70 were treated, 70 were not.[8] The trial was also fairly short by current standards: around a year and a half long. Table 1.1 is the tally sheet showing the number of participants who had bad health events (what we call outcomes) over that period—separated by whether they were randomized to the No Treatment group or the Treatment group.[9]

TABLE 1.1 *Outcomes in the VA Randomized Trial of Treatment for Severe Hypertension*

| Outcome | No Treatment (Control) | Treatment (Intervention) |
|---|---|---|
| Death | 4 | 0 |
| Stroke | 4 | 1 |
| Heart failure | 4 | 0 |
| Heart attack | 2 | 0 |
| Kidney failure | 3 | 0 |
| Eye hemorrhage | 7 | 0 |
| Hospitalized for high blood pressure | 3 | 0 |
| Treatment complication | 0 | 1 |
| **Total** | 27 | 2 |

Small study, short follow-up—yet powerful results. You see an awful lot of zeros in the Treatment group. And the bottom line is stark: 27 bad events in the No Treatment group versus 2 in the Treatment group.

To see how powerful this is, consider that there are a total of 29 participants who had bad events. If treatment made no difference, you'd expect the 29 events to be roughly split between the two groups. Now imagine flipping a coin 29 times and getting heads 27 times and tails only 2. What are the chances of that? If it's a fair coin, about two in a million. In other words, there is almost no way to get a difference like this in two similar groups (groups created by randomization) unless the treatment worked.

It is important to point out just how common these bad events were in the No Treatment group. Among 70 patients, 27 had something bad happen over the course of a year and a half. People don't usually think about the likelihood of any particular event happening over a period of 1.5 years (or, for that matter, over 3.3 or 4.7 years); we usually think about the chance of something happening over one year. The one-year chance of one of these bad events happening was about 26 percent. In other words, more than a quarter of the men with untreated severe diastolic hypertension had something very bad happen within one year (bad like a stroke, heart attack, or death). The corresponding risk for the Treatment group was less than 2 percent. There's a huge difference between 26 percent and less than 2 percent. It means that the treatment really helped. This is about as good as it gets in medicine. If I had severe diastolic hypertension, I'd definitely want to be diagnosed and treated.

Because most people with hypertension get treated for years, it helps to take a longer view into the future. You're probably concerned about strokes, heart attacks, and death not only for the next year but also for a longer time period. Looking at just the one-year time frame minimizes the risks you face; risks accumulate over time. So doctors often look at the chances of people experiencing bad health events over five or ten years. Based on the above data and assuming the rate of bad events is constant, the five-year risk of something bad happening to a person in the No Treatment group is around 80 percent. (For those wondering why it would not be more than 100 percent, remember that as time passes—and more bad events happen—fewer and fewer men are available to experience a first event. After five years, 80 percent of men with untreated severe diastolic hypertension have experienced a bad health event; after ten years, 95 percent; and after fifteen years, 99 percent. Now you see why I'm so sure that Mr. Lemay probably would have died years ago had he not been treated.)

Of course, the risk accumulates in the Treatment group as well: over five years, the likelihood of a bad event is 8 percent; over ten years, it's 15 percent, and over fifteen years, it's 21 percent.

So we can compare No Treatment versus Treatment using different amounts of time:

After five years, the chance of a bad event is 80 percent for the No Treatment group versus 8 percent for the Treatment group

or

After ten years, the chance of a bad event is 95 percent for the No Treatment group versus 15 percent for the Treatment group

or

After fifteen years, the chance of a bad event is 99 percent for the No Treatment group versus 21 percent for the Treatment group.

Regardless of which comparison you choose to look at, my guess is that you would choose treatment. I know I would.

There are other ways to think about the benefit. Let's stick with the five-year time frame. If you are not treated, you have an 80 percent chance of something bad happening over that period. If you are treated, that chance falls to 8 percent. So the likelihood that you will benefit from treatment—that is, avoid something bad because you have received treatment—is 72 percent (80 percent – 8 percent). And here's one more way to think about it. If one person has a 72 percent chance of benefiting, that means we need to treat fewer than two people (on average) to make sure one person will benefit. The exact number of patients we must treat is simply the reciprocal (or 1 divided by the number) of the chance of benefit. In this case, the number we want the reciprocal of is 72 percent, which is 0.72 in decimal form. The reciprocal of 0.72 is 1 divided by 0.72 (a calculator is handy here): 1.3888, which for simplicity's sake I'll round up to 1.4. Doctors call this the "number needed to treat": we need to treat an average of only 1.4 patients for five years to be sure that one person will benefit.

Table 1.2 summarizes these three ways to think about benefit.

TABLE 1.2  *Measures of Benefit*

| Measure | Definition | Example [Severe Diastolic Hypertension] |
|---|---|---|
| Five-year risk in each group | The chance of having a bad event in each group over five years | No Treatment group: 80 percent Treatment group: 8 percent |
| Chance of benefit (over five years) | Subtraction of the risk in the Treatment group from the risk in the No Treatment group = the chance of being helped by treatment | 80 percent – 8 percent: 72 percent of people benefit from treatment |
| Number needed to treat (over five years) | The reciprocal of the chance of benefit; the number of people that must be treated to ensure that one person benefits | 1 / 0.72 ≈ 1.4 people |

### Benefit across the spectrum of hypertension

The benefit of treating very high blood pressure—severe hypertension—is great. But hypertension varies in degrees of severity, from almost normal blood pressure to very high. And the benefit of treatment is affected by the degree of hypertension. I'd like to examine the benefit of treatment for different degrees of hypertension.

Table 1.3 shows the results of multiple randomized trials, each one looking at a different degree of hypertension.

TABLE 1.3  *Benefit across the Spectrum of Hypertension*

| Degree of Hypertension | Five-year Risk of Bad Event | | Chance of Benefit | Number Needed to Treat |
|---|---|---|---|---|
| | No Treatment | Treatment | | |
| Severe [Diastolic BP 115–129] | 80% | 8% | 72% | 1.4 |
| Moderate[10] [Diastolic BP 105–114] | 38% | 12% | 26% | 4 |
| Mild [Diastolic BP 90–104] | 32% | 23% | 9% | 11 |
| Very Mild[11] [Diastolic BP 90–100] | 9% | 3% | 6% | 18[12] |

Each successive row represents a study of patients with a progressively milder degree of hypertension (that is, lower diastolic blood pressures) than the preceding group. For each study, I made sure that a bad event meant roughly the same thing: death or serious problems with body organs (for example, a heart attack, a stroke, kidney failure). Note that in the No Treatment group (the second column), the likelihood of having a bad event falls as the level of blood pressure falls. This reflects a basic principle: *milder abnormalities are less likely to cause problems than severe abnormalities are.* You might have guessed that. But it's really an important point to remember. And you may even need to remind your doctor about it.

The third column is a little surprising. You might think that all the numbers should be about the same, that all people who are treated will end up with the same chance of a bad event. But these are real data, and real data aren't as tidy as we would like. These numbers bounce around a bit, probably reflecting differences in the patients studied and the drugs used—plus the fact that different studies will always produce somewhat different answers. So all of these numbers are only an approximation of the truth. The point is the big picture.

The chance that you will benefit from treatment (the fourth column) falls as the degree of hypertension becomes milder. This reflects a second basic principle: *people with milder abnormalities stand to benefit less from treatment than those with severe abnormalities.* The fifth column is another way of saying the same thing. While almost everyone treated for severe hypertension will benefit, eighteen people with mild hypertension have to be treated for one to benefit.

Because the second principle is so important in understanding the remainder of this book, I think it's useful to illustrate it with the drawing in figure 1.2:

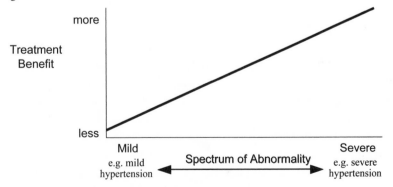

FIGURE 1.2 *Relationship between the Spectrum of the Abnormality and Treatment Benefit in Hypertension*

The bottom of the drawing shows the spectrum of the abnormality. Most conditions, like hypertension, exist on a spectrum: from very mild to severe forms. In general, treatment benefit rises with the severity of the abnormality. Of course, the two principles above are closely related. The reason people with milder abnormalities stand to benefit less from treatment is that milder abnormalities are less likely to cause problems (symptoms or death) than severe abnormalities. In other words, milder abnormalities are more likely to represent cases of overdiagnosis. Most people are not destined to have anything bad happen to them as a result of their mild abnormalities. And those who are overdiagnosed cannot benefit from treatment—there's nothing to fix.

At this point you might be thinking, *So what? If there's any chance of benefit, why not take the medication?* One reason is money. Some people have to spend a lot of their income on these medications; in order to afford the medicine, sometimes they'll have to spend less on necessities, such as food. Another reason not to take the medications is what I call the hassle factors: you have to make appointments with your doctor, get your prescriptions filled, get lab tests, make phone calls for refills, and fill out insurance forms. And finally, all other things being equal, some people prefer not to have to take daily medication.

But let's take all these reasons off the table. Suppose treatment is free, there's no hassle involved in getting it, and you are perfectly happy to take a daily medication. In that case, everybody would want to be treated, regardless of the severity of his or her hypertension and regardless of how small the benefit, right?

Unless, of course, there were downsides, some sort of harm associated with treatment.

### When the treatment is worse than the disease

Most of my clinical work has not involved the care of inpatients (patients in the hospital), but the care of outpatients (patients in the clinic). Many of the regular patients I see in clinic might be described as old-time Vermonters—rugged, elderly men who have spent most of their lives outdoors. (And because I work for the Department of Veterans Affairs, all of my patients have spent some portion of their lives in the military.) One such patient, Mr. Bailey, is an eighty-two-year-old man who lives alone on a farm about twenty-five miles away from the hospital. He spends most days working outdoors: clearing brush, tapping maple trees, shoveling snow, rebuilding stone walls, tending livestock, or fixing his house. I can't reach him on the phone unless

I call him after dark. (Adding to the challenge is the fact he doesn't have an answering machine.)

Luckily I haven't had to contact Mr. Bailey much, because he has been fairly healthy. Over the past decade, we have seen each other in clinic once or twice a year, and mostly we just talk. Honestly, I haven't done much for him. He's never been admitted to the hospital. The only regular medicine I've given him is for benign prostatic hypertrophy—a common condition in middle-aged and elderly men in which the prostate enlarges, compresses the urethra (the tube that drains the bladder), and interferes with the normal flow of urine (much like a clamp on a garden hose). We have contemplated treatment for his intermittent depression, but it has never been severe enough for me to argue strongly for it. Moreover, he has never been inclined to take medicine for it. He's fairly conservative about medical intervention in general.

It's probably worth digressing here to say that, although many of my patients actively seek medical intervention (believing that medical care can only help them feel better), a substantial portion of my patients fall into Mr. Bailey's category. They avoid elective surgery. They are hesitant about taking medicines for what they perceive to be minor problems. And they are predisposed to be skeptical about preventive interventions, interventions for conditions that aren't problems now but might become so in the future. I call it the "if it ain't broke, don't fix it" school of thought. I attribute their membership in this school to the fierce independent streak of many rural Vermonters—they are raised to be self-reliant (and may have regretted excessive mechanical interventions on their tractors).

A couple of winters ago, Mr. Bailey's name appeared on a list given to me by clinic administrators identifying which of my patients had blood pressures that the VA considered somehow suboptimal. His diastolic blood pressure had been fine, in the 70 to 90 range. But his systolic blood pressure had been high at his last two visits—both measurements in the 160s. Honestly, I can't tell you whether or not I knew this before I got the list. When I was in medical school, treatment decisions were based solely on the diastolic blood pressure. Now there is a growing recognition that among older individuals, systolic blood pressure elevations are probably more important than diastolic blood pressure elevations. I most likely saw the high systolic readings and simply didn't have any reaction. But now it was clear somebody else knew about them and had reacted.

I'd like to tell you that this fact in and of itself wouldn't influence my practice. But I can't. No doctor wants to be identified as being out of step with practice norms. I had mixed feelings about the importance of treating his mild systolic hypertension—I could make an argument either way. But seeing Mr. Bailey's name on the list was enough to get me to pursue treatment.

So I started Mr. Bailey on one twenty-five-milligram tablet of hydrochlorothiazide every morning. Hydrochlorothiazide is a diuretic: it makes a person urinate more, which lowers the amount of fluid in the body (part of the reason it lowers blood pressure). Mr. Bailey had no ill effects from the medicine. His blood pressure came down and was normal throughout the spring. Then we had a spell of hot, humid weather. That sort of thing doesn't stop Mr. Bailey. One day he was outside rebuilding a stone wall, lifting heavy rocks and dripping with sweat. And since he's not the kind of guy to tote a water bottle around with him, he got dehydrated. His blood pressure got too low and he collapsed.

When he woke up, he called me. (I'm easier to get on the phone than he is.) He hadn't hurt himself when he fainted, but he could have. And what if he had been using his chain saw? I told him to stop the medicine, drink more water, and see me in clinic.

When I saw him a few days later, he seemed fine. I told him that I suspected that the combination of sweating, not drinking water, and the blood pressure medicine had made him faint. He wanted to know whether he really had to take the medicine at all. A perfectly reasonable question. Because I'm a researcher, I thought I'd look for some numbers so he could consider the question more carefully.

While the treatment of diastolic hypertension dates back to the 1960s, the treatment of systolic hypertension is much more recent. The study that changed our practice was a randomized trial published in 1991.[13] The trial enrolled elderly patients (like Mr. Bailey) whose diastolic blood pressures were normal but whose systolic blood pressures were over 160, a condition called isolated systolic hypertension. The study was big—almost five thousand patients. And the follow-up was long—almost five years. For those familiar with clinical research, these details are a clue about the size of the effect researchers expected to find. Remember the VA randomized trial? It was a small study with a short follow-up that found a huge effect. If a huge effect exists, it will be found using a small number of people in a short amount of time. If a study is really large and has a long follow-up, that's a clue that the effect the researchers are looking for is small.

In the study of isolated systolic hypertension, the researchers were looking for the same outcomes that were found in studies of diastolic hypertension: death and problems stemming from damage to the blood vessels supplying the heart and brain. Because the patients in the study were relatively old (in their seventies and eighties), these events were fairly common in the No Treatment group—18 percent had bad events over five years. The Treatment group did somewhat better—13 percent had bad events over five years.

I shared the numbers with Mr. Bailey. Since the life expectancy of an eighty-two-year-old white male is about seven years,[14] the five-year time frame seemed appropriate. I told him the chance of something bad happening in the next five years was 18 percent without treatment and 13 percent with treatment. That means 5 percent of patients will benefit from treatment (18 – 13). Twenty patients will have to be treated for one to benefit (1 / 0.05). He was perplexed. To him, the benefit seemed really small. Why on earth would he choose treatment?

No sale. Mr. Bailey didn't focus on the possibility that he might be the one person in twenty who benefited. He worried he would be one of nineteen who did not. He was worried about overdiagnosis. And he had a problem with the medication now; he had already experienced a harmful side effect. He chose not to be treated.[15] Perfectly rational.

■   ■   ■

THE MANAGEMENT OF HYPERTENSION REPRESENTED a true paradigm shift in medicine: from treating patients experiencing health problems now to treating people who may develop problems in the future. It marked the beginning of treatment for people without symptoms—people who felt well but who were more likely than the average person to develop disease.

While treatment does save lives, it doesn't save everyone's life. It doesn't prevent every heart attack and stroke. And some people with hypertension aren't destined to experience these problems even without treatment. They face a different problem: overdiagnosis. There are downsides to being treated for hypertension, some more serious than others. I don't want to overemphasize the physical side effects of medical treatment, but they are there. Some medicines can cause fatigue, others can cause cough, still others can impair sex drive. All of them can make your blood pressure too low, leading to light-headedness, fainting, and falls. And for the elderly, major falls can be the start of a chain of events that lead to death. The balance between the potential benefit of treatment and the risk of overdiagnosis is closely related to where a person falls on the abnormality spectrum—in other words, how high his or her blood pressure is—and to how aggressively we choose to lower it.[16] If you have severe hypertension (systolic or diastolic), treatment is a no-brainer. But as the degree of hypertension falls, the decision to treat becomes a much tougher call. And theoretically, at least, there is some point where the benefit of treatment is so small and the chance of overdiagnosis so high that the decision once again becomes a no-brainer: there's simply no point to diagnosis and treatment.

This raises the question: Where should we draw the line? In other words, when should something be considered a condition that warrants treatment?

# CHAPTER 2

# We Change the Rules

*How Numbers Get Changed to Give You Diabetes,*
*High Cholesterol, and Osteoporosis*

AS YOU SAW IN THE previous chapter, hypertension is defined by a numerical rule. If your blood pressure is above a certain number, you have hypertension. If it isn't above that number, you don't. But hypertension isn't the only condition defined by a numerical rule. There are many conditions that you can be labeled with simply because you are on the wrong side of a number, not because you have any symptoms. Diabetes is defined by a number for blood sugar; hyperlipidemia is defined by a number for cholesterol; and osteoporosis is defined by a number for bone density (called a T score). Of course, in each of these conditions doctors are trying to get ahead of symptoms—we are trying to make diagnoses early in order to prevent bad events such as leg amputation and blindness from diabetes, heart attacks and strokes from high cholesterol, and wrist and hip fractures from osteoporosis. But whenever we make diagnoses ahead of symptoms, overdiagnosis becomes a problem. Some people diagnosed with diabetes, high cholesterol, and osteoporosis will never develop symptoms or die from the conditions. And this is most likely the case for those in whom the condition is mild.

The numerical rules used to define conditions are really important. They typically involve a single number: if you fall on one side of the number you are defined as well; if you're on the other, you are defined as abnormal. These numbers—called cutoffs or thresholds—determine who has a condition and who doesn't. They determine who gets treatment and who doesn't. And they determine how much overdiagnosis occurs.

Cutoffs are set by expert panels of physicians. I wish I could say that their determinations result from purely scientific processes. But they are more haphazard than that: they involve value judgments, and even financial interests. The experts who select the cutoffs have particular sets of beliefs about what is important. Because these doctors care greatly about the conditions they specialize in, I believe they sometimes lose a broader perspective. Their focus is to do everything they can to avoid the bad events associated with the condition; their main concern is not missing anyone who could possibly benefit from diagnosis and treatment. So they tend to set cutoffs that are expansive, leading many to be labeled abnormal. They tend to either ignore or downplay the major pitfall of this strategy: treating those who will not benefit.

Over the past few decades many cutoffs have been changed in a way that dramatically increases the number of individuals who are labeled with these conditions. It means that the threshold to make a diagnosis has fallen. Even if this is done with the best of intentions—to avoid more bad events—it can lead to an undesirable consequence: more overdiagnosis.

### How bad things happen when we try to do good

This is not a happy story. Mr. Roberts was a seventy-four-year-old man whose major medical problem was ulcerative colitis—an inflammatory condition of his colon (the large intestine). It's a disease that causes symptoms such as severe abdominal pain and diarrhea (and it also increases the risk of colon cancer). Because his disease was so severe, he had part of his colon surgically removed. Although this led him to have frequent bowel movements, he learned to deal with his situation quite well.

One day, in a routine lab test, Mr. Roberts was found to have an elevated blood sugar. It wasn't that high, but the finding prompted more testing. And more testing confirmed the diagnosis: diabetes. He had type 2 diabetes—the form of the disease that typically occurs in older adults (as opposed to type 1, which usually starts in childhood). Although he had no symptoms of diabetes, over the past few decades doctors had gotten much more aggressive about treating it early, so his primary care physician started him on glyburide—a drug that lowers blood sugar. The medication worked well.

Six months later he blacked out while driving on the local interstate. His car went off the road and rolled over. He fractured his sixth and seventh cervical vertebrae—in other words, he broke his neck. The paramedics on the scene measured his blood sugar. It was very low. The medication had worked *too* well. I'd hate to have been the doctor who prescribed him glyburide.

But I was that doctor. I'm not sure what happened. I had used the standard starting dose of medication. He had tolerated it well for almost half a year. Maybe he hadn't eaten normally that day; maybe he had the flu, or some stomach virus. I don't know.

Mr. Roberts was in the hospital for over a month. When I next saw him in clinic he was wearing a halo brace. The halo is a metal ring that encircles the head, much like the brim of a hat, except the halo doesn't sit on the head—it is secured to the skull with pins. Attached to it are two metal rods that extend to the shoulders and are connected to a tightly fitted plastic jacket. With this apparatus, the neck is both immobilized and stretched so that the fracture can heal. I felt terrible. And—maybe it goes without saying—I didn't restart the glyburide.

Mr. Roberts is now ninety and is still a patient of mine. He has not been treated for diabetes since the accident, nor has he had any complications from diabetes. I think he was overdiagnosed. But he was lucky. There was no permanent injury. He has recovered fully from the problems caused by his unneeded treatment. But I'm not sure I have.

### Who has diabetes?

Diabetes can be a very serious disease. Some patients with the disease—usually children—first come to medical attention because they lose consciousness. They are in a diabetic coma: their blood sugar may be ten times normal, their potassium stores are extremely low, and their body fluids are dangerously acidic (we call it a metabolic acidosis). Without treatment, they die.

Treating a patient in a diabetic coma is one of the most rewarding experiences in medicine. The patient comes in near death, and generally about two days later he feels fine. All the patient needs is lots of intravenous fluids, some potassium, and the hormone that was lacking—insulin. Insulin is the hormone that allows sugar to move from the blood into the cells. Giving it, along with the fluid and potassium, normalizes the blood sugar and the acid-base balance. More important, the patient wakes up. It's really something to see.

But what I have just described is actually the less common form of diabetes—type 1. Patients with type 2, the much more common form, are usually adults and have plenty of insulin. Their problem is that the insulin doesn't work because the body has become resistant to it. These patients are frequently overweight (and the best treatment is losing weight). While it does not tend to lead to a diabetic coma, this type of diabetes can still be a very bad disease. Either type can lead to severe complications, including blindness, kidney failure, heart disease, impaired healing of wounds, and leg infections requiring amputation. But type 2 diabetes can also be a totally asymptomatic condition. So just like hypertension, there is a spectrum of abnormality in diabetes. Some people with the diagnosis will develop the aforementioned complications; others will not. Although we are never sure exactly who these others are, they have been overdiagnosed.

So how do we decide who has diabetes? When I was in medical school, our numerical rule was this: if you had a fasting blood sugar over 140, then you had diabetes. But in 1997 the Expert Committee on the Diagnosis and Classification of Diabetes Mellitus redefined the disorder.[1] Now if you have a fasting blood sugar over 126, you have diabetes. So everyone who has a blood sugar between 126 and 140 used to be normal but now has diabetes. That little change turned over 1.6 million people into patients.[2]

Is that a problem? Maybe, maybe not. Because we changed the rules, we now treat more patients for diabetes. That may mean that we have lowered the chance of diabetic complications for some of these new patients. But because these patients have milder diabetes (relatively low blood sugars between 126 and 140), they are at relatively low risk for these complications to begin with.

So just like people with relatively mild hypertension, people with mildly abnormal blood sugar levels have less to gain from treatment.

Figure 2.1 illustrates the effect of broadening the numbers defining diabetes—moving down the spectrum of the abnormality—on the benefit of treatment. My editor noticed that it's pretty much the same figure as the one in the first chapter. And, of course, it is. But that's the point. Furthermore, the relationship depicted in the figure applies equally well to the other disorders in this chapter: just replace the "mild diabetes" and "severe diabetes" poles of the spectrum with "near normal cholesterol" and "very high cholesterol" or "mild osteoporosis" and "severe osteoporosis," and you'll get the picture.

In fact, the relationship applies to all of medical care. As we expand treatment to people with progressively milder abnormalities, their potential to benefit from treatment becomes progressively smaller. So the redundancy is purposeful—I really want you to write this concept to your hard drive.

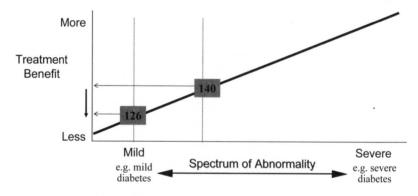

FIGURE 2.1 *Effect of Changing the Rules in Diabetes*

Severe abnormalities are different. Just like it's bad to have really high blood pressure, it's bad to have really high blood sugar. You want to take action to lower both. But remember: it's also bad to have a blood pressure that is too low. And it's bad to have a blood sugar that is too low—just ask Mr. Roberts.

The general problem was dramatically demonstrated in a recent random-ized trial from the National Institutes of Health.[3] The trial was designed to determine whether intensively lowering blood sugar reduced the risk of hav-ing or dying from a heart attack or stroke. The trial enrolled over ten thou-sand patients with diabetes at high risk for these events. About five thousand were randomized to receive standard diabetes therapy—therapy to lower their average blood sugar to a more acceptable, although not normal, range. The other five thousand were randomized to receive intensive drug ther-apy—therapy to make their blood sugar normal. And half of these patients achieved the goal: the average blood sugar level was below 140.[4] Because the average includes blood sugars measured right after eating (which tend to be high), it is safe to assume that their fasting blood sugars were considerably lower.

The trial started in 2003 and was supposed to continue to 2009. But on February 6, 2008, the National Heart, Blood, and Lung Institute issued a press release saying they were "changing" the intensive therapy regimen "due to safety concerns."[5] *Changing* wasn't the most accurate word to describe what they were doing; *stopping* would have been a better choice. And the safety concern was that patients receiving intensive therapy were dying more often than patients receiving standard therapy. After three years, 5 percent of patients receiving intensive therapy had died, compared with 4 percent of those receiving standard therapy. It was about a 25 percent in-crease in the risk of death, and the researchers were confident that it was not a statistical fluke. There was little doubt: intensive treatment was worse than standard treatment.

You might wonder how making people's blood sugar normal could end up killing them. It's probably because we can't simply dial a patient's blood sugar to a specific number; our therapies aren't that precise. Instead, blood sugar bounces around, and if we try to have blood sugar bounce around normal, sometimes it will bounce too low. And having your blood sugar too low increases your risk of death. The investigators might argue that hypoglyce-mia (low blood sugar) was not the cause of the increased risk of death. But by their own admission, they were not sure what explained the increased mortality. In the official report, lead author Hertzel C. Gerstein wrote: "De-spite detailed analyses, we have been unable to identify the precise cause of the increased risk of death in the intensive blood sugar strategy group . . . Our analyses to date suggest that no specific medication or com-bination of medications is responsible. We believe that some unidentified combination of factors tied to the overall medical strategy is likely at play." My view is that if the trial had shown a mortality benefit, the authors would have been quick to ascribe that benefit to intensive control of blood sugar (as I think would have been correct in that case). But since the trial showed a mortality harm, that must also be ascribed to intensive control of blood sugar. That's the point of a randomized trial.

What does this study tell us about where to set the threshold to diagnose diabetes? My take is this: if it's not good to make diabetics have near normal blood sugars, then it's not good to label those with near normal blood sugars diabetics. Why? Because doctors will treat them. People with mild blood sugar elevations are the least likely to gain from treatment—and arguably the most likely to be harmed, as Mr. Roberts was.

### Beyond diabetes

This isn't only about diabetes. The tendency to lower the threshold of diagnosis has been repeated in a number of other common conditions, including, as we've seen, hypertension. Prior to 1997, many physicians did not treat patients with mild hypertension. Although the Joint National Committee on High Blood Pressure recommended treating these individuals, they acknowledged that reasonable doctors might disagree with this recommendation "in the absence of target organ damage (e.g., no eye, kidney or heart problems) and other major risk factors, some physicians may elect to withhold antihypertensive drug therapy." But in 1997 the committee took a hard line and strongly advocated drug therapy for all patients with mild hypertension, regardless of their risk of cardiovascular disease.[6]

This stance effectively redefined hypertension requiring pharmacologic treatment. Diastolic blood pressures above 90 mm Hg (instead of 100) now required treatment. And systolic blood pressures above 140 mm Hg (instead of 160) now required treatment. This apparently small change had a big effect. It meant an additional thirteen million Americans met criteria for antihypertensive therapy.[7]

The same pattern played out with cholesterol. The definition of abnormal cholesterol has changed so often since I finished medical school that it is hard for me to keep track. The only thing that has been consistent is the direction of the change—always lower and lower thresholds to define cholesterol as abnormally high. Our bible in medical school was a book called *Harrison's Principles of Internal Medicine* (mine was the eighth edition; it is now in its seventeenth edition). It recommended that therapy be reserved for patients whose total cholesterol was over 300.

Soon the measurement of cholesterol got much more complex. We could measure various types of cholesterol: the low-density cholesterol (known as

LDL, the so-called bad cholesterol) and the high-density cholesterol (known as HDL, the so-called good cholesterol). Having subtyped cholesterol, we could develop ratios—LDL to HDL, LDL to total, and so forth. Recommendations were then tailored based on the other risk factors for heart disease (such as smoking, high blood pressure, a prior heart attack). While some of this made good sense—particularly being more aggressive in those who had already had heart attacks (for whom the benefit of lowering cholesterol is greatest)—it did result in a very complex set of recommendations.

Despite this complexity, by the mid-1990s large health-care organizations (such as the Department of Veterans Affairs, for whom I work) had settled on defining a total cholesterol above 240 as being abnormal and warranting therapy. But in 1998 a major randomized trial changed things. The Air Force / Texas Coronary Atherosclerosis Prevention Study demonstrated a reduction in what was called "first acute major coronary events" (a combination of fatal and nonfatal heart attacks, unstable angina, and sudden cardiac death) when what was then considered normal cholesterol was lowered from an average of 228 to 184. Over five years, about 5 percent of patients with untreated normal cholesterol had one of these events, while only 3 percent of patients with treated normal cholesterol did.[8] Thus the chance of benefit was 2 percent (5 percent − 3 percent).[9] So for every one hundred patients treated over five years, two were helped and ninety-eight were not.

All of a sudden the threshold for abnormal total cholesterol fell from greater than 240 to greater than 200. This change affected a lot of people—an additional forty-two million "new cases" of high cholesterol.[10] Forty-two million people—that's a big number. You might reasonably wonder why so many people were affected. Figure 2.2 shows the pattern of cholesterol levels in American adults (statisticians call this the distribution of cholesterol in the population). A cholesterol of 200 is almost right in the middle—just about average for the U.S. adult population. Moving the cutoff this close to the average has a huge effect on the number of people diagnosed.

You may have noticed something else in figure 2.2: there are a lot more people with cholesterol in the 200-to-240 range than there are in the 240-to-280 range. And there are more people with cholesterol levels in the 240-to-280 range than there are in the 280-to-320 range. In other words, mildly abnormal cholesterol levels are much more common than markedly abnormal cholesterol levels. This is true for every condition in this chapter. So an apparently small change in the cutoff can dramatically affect the number of people turned into patients. And as with diabetes and hypertension, people with mildly elevated cholesterol stand to benefit less from treatment than those with

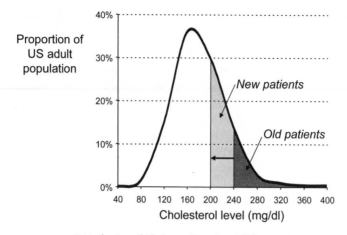

FIGURE 2.2  *Distribution of Cholesterol Level in Adult Americans and the Effect of Changing the Cutoff from 240 to 200*

severely elevated cholesterol. Lowering the cutoff for what is considered abnormal not only turns a large number of people into patients but also produces patients with the mildest form of the condition.

Then there's osteoporosis. My classmates and I didn't think much about the early diagnosis of osteoporosis in medical school. It was a clinical diagnosis reserved for patients experiencing symptoms, usually painful, spontaneous fractures of the back (vertebral compression fractures). Osteoporosis is often referred to colloquially as "thinning of the bones"; the literal meaning is that the bone (the *osteo-* prefix) becomes more porous. It's a process that that invariably occurs as we age, although it is more rapid in some than in others. Frankly, doctors didn't have a reliable way to measure this process, so we focused instead on its clinical consequences.

Then bone mineral density testing came along. It is an X-ray of a specific bone (usually the spine, hip, or wrist). But it's not used to see if the bone is broken; it is used to measure how dense the bone is—that is, how much bone is there.[11] The advent of this test allowed us to begin to quantify how dense people's bones were by using a T score. A T score quantifies the bone density of a patient compared to "normal"—which is defined as the average bone density of white women ages twenty to twenty-nine. (For this condition, women have historically been the focus.) If your bone density is the same as that of the typical twenty- to twenty-nine-year-old white woman—regardless of your own age and ethnicity—then your T score would be 0. If your bones are a whole lot denser than average, your T score could be as high as 3.[12] If your bones are a whole lot *thinner* than average, your T score could be as low as −3.

Negative numbers have a way of making things more difficult, so it is unfortunate that most women will have negative T scores. The reason is that most women who are tested for osteoporosis are considerably older than the group to which they are being compared. Because bones thin with age, older women generally have thinner bones than younger women. Thus, their T scores are typically less than 0. The World Health Organization originally defined osteoporosis as a T score of less than −2.5. It was an arbitrary number to pick. But they were correct in saying that women with T scores of less than −2.5 (farther from zero, for example, −2.8) are at higher risk for fracture than women with T scores greater than −2.5 (closer to zero, for example, −2.2). Of course, this could be said about any cutoff: women with T scores less than 0 are at higher risk than women with T scores above 0, women with T scores less than −1 are at higher risk than women with T scores above −1, and so on.

Perhaps recognizing this, the National Osteoporosis Foundation in 2003 advocated treating all women with T scores of less than −2.0 for osteoporosis. The argument for expanding the definition was based on the observation that most hip fractures occurred in women whose bone densities were above a T score of −2.5. Now, you wouldn't think the difference between −2.5 and −2.0—a measly 0.5—would matter that much. But given what you've learned about cholesterol, you might guess that mildly abnormal T scores are more common than markedly abnormal T scores. So perhaps you won't be surprised to hear that literally overnight, 6.7 million American women developed osteoporosis.[13]

Four conditions; four changes in the thresholds used to diagnose them. Table 2.1 summarizes what has happened.

TABLE 2.1  *Effect of Lower Diagnostic Thresholds on the Number of "Diseased" Americans*

| Condition | Disease Prevalence | | | |
|---|---|---|---|---|
| Change in Threshold | Old Definition | New Definition | **New Cases** | **Increase** |
| Diabetes<br>Fasting sugar 140 → 126 | 11,697,000 | 13,378,000 | 1,681,000 | 14% |
| Hypertension<br>Systolic BP 160 → 140<br>Diastolic BP 100 → 90 | 38,690,000 | 52,180,000 | 13,490,000 | 35% |
| Hyperlipidemia<br>Total cholesterol 240 → 200 | 49,480,000 | 92,127,000 | 42,647,000 | 86% |
| Osteoporosis in women<br>T score −2.5 → −2.0 | 8,010,000 | 14,791,000 | 6,781,000 | 85% |

You can see how changing cutoffs dramatically increased the number of people labeled with the conditions (and who were then said to need treatment). Whether or not that was a good thing for the affected individuals is a tough question. But there's no question about whether or not it was a good thing for business. These changes substantially increased the market for treatments—and the money to be made from them.

There are widespread concerns about the independence of the experts who set the cutoffs for all of the conditions we have discussed. The head of the diabetes cutoff panel was a paid consultant to Aventis Pharmaceuticals, Bristol-Myers Squibb, Eli Lilly, GlaxoSmithKline, Novartis, Merck, and Pfizer—all of which make diabetes drugs.[14] Nine of the eleven authors of recent high blood pressure guidelines had some kind of financial ties—as paid consultants, paid speakers, or grant recipients—to drug companies that made high blood pressure drugs.[15] Similarly, eight of the nine experts who lowered the cholesterol cutoff were paid consultants to drug companies making cholesterol drugs.[16] And the first cutoff for osteoporosis was established by a World Health Organization panel in partnership with the International Osteoporosis Foundation—an organization whose corporate advisory board consisted of thirty-one drug and medical equipment companies.[17]

To be fair, many of these experts may be true believers, people who want to do everything they can not to miss anyone who could possibly benefit from diagnosis. But the fact that there is so much money on the table may lead them to overestimate the benefits and ignore the harms of overdiagnosis. These decisions affect too many people to let them be tainted by the businesses that stand to gain from them.

### Problems with treatment

But let's say you don't care that cutoffs may have been lowered merely to make money. So what if doctors have expanded the definitions of these conditions and turned millions of Americans into patients? Some of these patients are destined to develop disease—symptoms, complications, and even death. And some fraction of these (but not all) can be helped by treatment initiated because of early diagnosis. No question about it—that's good, you might think.

But as a group, the additional patients diagnosed because of the lowered thresholds have the mildest abnormalities of any patients with the condition. They are at the lowest risk to develop the bad events associated with their conditions. So while some are destined to develop problems, most are not—they have been overdiagnosed and can only be harmed by diagnosis and treatment. This is the tension we will keep coming back to throughout this book. A few may be helped, a lot will be overdiagnosed, and some of them will be harmed. And no one knows who is in which group.

The conventional ethos of medicine has been to focus on the potential benefit for the few and to downplay the rest. So the medical experts search for those who are plausibly at higher risk and then suggest that the rest of us doctors should identify and treat them. But consider the best data to use when thinking about the trade-off: the data from the randomized trials.

For cholesterol, the previously mentioned Air Force / Texas Coronary Atherosclerosis Prevention Study is a good example. You will recall that it studied the effects of lowering near normal cholesterol levels (levels between 200 and 240) in people without heart disease. Let's first focus on the people whose cholesterol was not treated (people randomized to the placebo group). Over five years, 5 percent of untreated patients had their first major heart events.

To get a sense of how much overdiagnosis happens, we need an estimate of the chance of an event occurring over a lifetime. That reflects the ultimate criterion for overdiagnosis: at the end of life, if the person never developed a problem from her condition, she has been overdiagnosed. To calculate the chance over a lifetime, I extrapolated the five-year experience to twenty-four years (the life expectancy of a fifty-eight-year-old, the average age of the people in the trial). This approach produces the following estimate: 22 percent of untreated patients in the trial would be expected to experience a first major heart event in their lifetimes. That means the other 78 percent were overdiagnosed.

You may be wondering how well treatment works over a lifetime (because cholesterol medicines are prescribed for a lifetime). After twenty-four years (if the benefit in the study persists), 14 percent of treated patients will have had a first major heart event (as compared with 22 percent of the untreated patients). That means only 8 percent would have been helped by treatment (22 − 14, the chance-of-benefit calculation).

So, given these estimates, here's the deal for near normal cholesterol.

---

If one hundred patients are diagnosed with near normal cholesterol
and treated for a lifetime, how many will be . . .

**Winners**
(treatment saved them from first major heart events)                                      8

**Treated for Naught**
(had first major heart events despite treatment)                                          14

**Losers**
(overdiagnosed—treatment couldn't help them because they were
never going to have heart events)                                                         78

---

Diagnose and treat a hundred patients, and eight of them are winners—they are helped by treatment because they avoid a first major heart event. For fourteen of them the effort was all for naught—they have their first major heart events despite treatment (they are not overdiagnosed, but they are also not helped, and they may have experienced side effects from treatment). The remaining seventy-eight are losers—they have been overdiagnosed. Even without treatment, none was going to have a heart attack.

Here are the same calculations for osteoporosis, using the data from another randomized trial: the Fracture Intervention Trial.[18] It studied the effect of increasing near normal bone density in women who had not had fractures previously. Over four years, 14 percent of untreated patients had symptomatic fractures. Extrapolating to an eighteen-year period (the life expectancy of the typical woman in the trial, a sixty-eight-year-old), 49 percent of untreated women would have gotten fractures.

That means 51 percent were overdiagnosed.

How does this treatment work over a lifetime? After eighteen years (if the benefit found in the study persists), 44 percent of treated women will have had fractures (as compared with 49 percent of untreated women). So only 5 percent are helped by treatment (49 – 44).

So here's the deal for near normal bone density.

---

If one hundred patients are diagnosed with near normal osteoporosis and treated for a lifetime, how many will be . . .

**Winners**
(treatment saved them from a fracture)                                      5

**Treated for Naught**
(had fractures despite treatment)                                          44

**Losers**
(overdiagnosed—treatment couldn't help them because they were
never going to have fractures)                                             51

---

Diagnose and treat a hundred patients, and five of them are winners—they are helped because they avoid fractures. For forty-four of them the effort was all for naught—they have bad events despite treatment (they are not overdiagnosed, but they are also not helped, and they may have experienced side effects from treatment). The remaining fifty-one are losers—they have been overdiagnosed.

Would you take the deal or would you pass? There's no right answer. It's a tough call.

You might say, Why not take it? Well, there are really good reasons to avoid being overdiagnosed with diabetes and hypertension: you don't want either your blood sugar or your blood pressure to go too low. Is it bad to have a cholesterol level that's too low? We don't think so now, but we don't have any long-term data on this question. Some scientists are concerned because the human body needs some cholesterol to build and repair cells. The commonly used medications to lower cholesterol—the class of drugs called statins—are generally very safe. Sometimes a new one is withdrawn for health concerns (so try to stick with the old ones), and they all have a tiny risk of a big problem: the rapid breakdown of muscles. But by and large they are as good as medicines get—particularly for preventing a second heart attack.

Is it bad to have too high a bone density? I'd say probably not. But I'm even less sure of this since we have less experience with the commonly used medications to increase bone density, the class of drugs called bisphosphonates. There is some concern about the long-term effects of these drugs; they may actually make bones more brittle by changing the bone architecture. They can also disturb calcium metabolism, lead to ulcers in the esophagus, and, very rarely, cause bone to die.[19] Hopefully we'll know more with longer-term studies.

But the real downside of accepting all these changes in the rules of diagnosis is that it is a slippery slope that is turning more and more of us into patients. Too many of us are already on too many medications. To be sure, some people may feel safer having their potential problems diagnosed and treated. For some, that may make the treatment side effects and hassle factors seem worth it. But this sense of being safer is partly the product of powerful messages that have systematically overstated the benefits of the diagnosis and treatment of mild abnormalities (and largely said nothing about the potential harms). Thus, the sense of being safer is likely an exaggerated view of the reality.

### And there's more to come

In 1997, the Joint National Committee on High Blood Pressure considered the creation of a new disease category: high-normal blood pressure, which would include people whose diastolic blood pressures ranged between 85 and 89 or whose systolic blood pressures ranged between 130 and 139. Then about ten years later, high-normal blood pressure got a new name: prehypertension. A large randomized trial demonstrated that giving people with prehypertension medicines to lower blood pressure reduced their chances of going on to develop hypertension.[20] (Why am I not surprised? Of course taking blood pressure medications lowers blood pressure!)

The first two years of the randomized trial compared a Treatment group (using a drug called candesartan) versus a No Treatment group (using placebos). At the end of the two-year period, 14 percent had developed hypertension in the Treatment group, while 40 percent had developed hypertension in the No Treatment group. That's a big difference—particularly when expressed as a "66 percent reduction" in developing hypertension. But of course this is going to happen—giving a drug that lowers blood pressure will indeed lower people's blood pressure and prevent many from developing hypertension. It tells you nothing about whether they benefit from the drug.

To be fair, the study did ask a second question. For the second two years, the randomized trial continued by giving both groups placebos. At the end of the four-year period, 53 percent of people in the group that had received treatment for two years had developed hypertension versus 63 percent of people in the group that had never received treatment. I'll admit—that's more interesting. It looks like treating for two years and then stopping leads to less hypertension than not treating at all. But the effect is small. And the bigger question remains: is it useful to prevent hypertension by treating the condition before it occurs? Why not wait and treat only those who develop hypertension? The important issue is whether treating prehypertension helps people avoid heart attacks, strokes, and deaths. We don't know whether treating prehypertension changes anybody's risk of heart attack, stroke, or death. But we do know that it's an enormous market—about eighteen million new patients.[21]

In 2002, the American Diabetes Association coined the term *prediabetes*—blood sugar levels that are higher than normal but not yet high enough to be diagnosed as diabetes. They said (and I have no reason to question this) that there were fifty-seven million people in the United States who had prediabetes.[22] That's an even bigger market, with huge ramifications for overdiagnosis and overtreatment. And low-cholesterol advocates are also looking to expand their condition: now they argue we should test children. The American Academy of Pediatrics says doctors should be performing cholesterol screening in kids who are overweight or who have parents with heart disease or high cholesterol. Because so many parents are diagnosed with high cholesterol, this will affect a lot of kids. Screening is supposed to start sometime before age ten (but after age two). Drug treatment is supposed to wait until age eight.[23]

To their credit, the National Osteoporosis Foundation experts have refined their guidelines for treating that disease. They have expanded the T score cutoff for treatment to −1.0, but they are clear that this by itself is not enough to warrant treatment. A patient should also have a greater than 3 percent chance of fracturing a hip in the next ten years.[24] This probability is calculated using a WHO algorithm that has been adapted for the United States. That algorithm requires doctors to go to a Web site and enter the patient's age, weight, height, and T score. It also requires data about whether the patient smokes; uses steroid medications; has a prior history of fracture, rheumatoid arthritis, or any disorder strongly associated with osteoporosis; or has three or more alcoholic drinks per day. If the doctor scrolls down, he or she will find detailed definitions of each of these risk factors, which the doctor needs to understand before interviewing the patient. The doctor then interviews the patient and enters the data into the algorithm, and the computer then does a series of calculations to determine the patient's chance of having a hip fracture in the next ten years.[25] If the number is higher than 3 percent, treatment is suggested.

It's a step forward in terms of better defining who is at high risk. But we really don't know whether this refinement helps because treatment hasn't been evaluated in women who have other risk factors in conjunction with a nearly normal bone density (for example, a T score of –1.0). Furthermore, the recommendation is complex enough—and sufficiently time consuming—that I wonder if many physicians won't simply default to treating every woman with a T score less than –1.0. That would mean virtually all older women. And now there is a movement for treating osteoporosis in men . . .

### Cascade of events

One of my neighbors has a good friend who lives outside of New York City. Lara regularly comes north to Vermont to escape the city, so I've gotten to know her over the years. She's a healthy sixty-five-year-old woman who nonetheless has managed to get entangled in quite a cascade of diagnosis and intervention. It started when Lara was screened for osteoporosis almost a decade ago. Her bone mineral density test showed that her T score was –1.8. Even though no one calls that osteoporosis (yet), her primary care doctor told her that she was at risk for fracture even though she had none of the aforementioned risk factors. (In this sense, we are all at risk.) She was also told that treatment was both easy and effective.

She told me that her reaction at the time was *Why not?* So she was started on hormone replacement therapy, which has been shown to increase bone density and reduce the chance of fracture. She tolerated the medicine well. Then along came the major randomized trials of hormone replacement therapy that confirmed its beneficial effects on bone strength but also demonstrated harmful effects—an increased risk of heart attacks and stroke, and an increased risk of breast cancer. Her doctor suggested she not take the medicine anymore and instead try a different medication for osteoporosis.

Lara was started on one of the bisphosphonates and did all right—for a while. Then she developed terrible pain when swallowing. She was referred to a gastroenterologist, who performed an endoscopy (a procedure in which a fiber-optic scope is passed through the mouth into the stomach) and found that she had severe inflammation and ulcers in her esophagus—a known side effect of bisphosphonates. She was switched to another medicine. The esophagitis healed, but a painful rash appeared all over her body. So she was referred to a dermatologist, who suspected that the rash was due to the medication. The medication was stopped, and the rash went away.

Lara had become a medical challenge because doctors couldn't figure out how to treat her. She was referred to an endocrinologist. Because osteoporosis is considered an endocrine disorder, endocrinologists are thought to be the experts in its treatment; just the people to send the osteoporosis patient who is a medical challenge.

Lest you forget, Lara didn't even have osteoporosis. At worst, she had osteopenia (you can think of that as preosteoporosis). And she didn't have any of the risk factors that would make a fracture more likely. Ideally the specialist would rethink the most fundamental question: is this a condition that warrants treatment? Based on Lara's T score and the absence of other fracture risk factors, her chances of having a fracture were low; consequently, the benefit of treatment would be small at best.

But the endocrinologist didn't raise this point; he was dealing with a medical challenge. So he conducted a thorough evaluation of all her glands and hormones. The evaluation included a careful physical exam of the thyroid gland, during which the endocrinologist thought he felt a lump. Lara was referred to a radiologist, who did an ultrasound exam of the thyroid and who found three lumps (the largest of which was about an inch in diameter). She had needles stuck in all of them and some fluid removed from each. Some of the cells in the fluid looked concerning under the microscope. The pathologist worried that they might be cancer, but the only way to know for sure was to remove her thyroid. So she was referred to a surgeon.

Imagine that. You feel fine, but someone suggests a test to see how strong your bones are. The test shows your density is just a little below average for your age. But you are considered at risk for fracture and encouraged to take action. Three medications and three specialists later, you are told you might have thyroid cancer. Quite a cascade. At least there's a happy ending in this case. A surgeon—I would say a prudent one—put a stop to it. He knew that virtually all adults have some evidence of thyroid cancer. Most important, Lara is fine—I just saw her kayaking on the Connecticut River—but now she's a little more hesitant to look for things to be wrong.

I can't tell you how often these diagnosis-and-treatment cascades occur—no one keeps tabs on this sort of thing. But I can tell you that, while they won't happen to most people, they are not that uncommon. It's another downside to becoming a patient prematurely.

■ ■ ■

IT IS EASY TO MAKE an argument that rules should be changed and numbers altered to redefine what is considered abnormal. There is always a case to be made that doing so could conceivably help a few more people. The discussion typically ends there. But even small changes can turn millions of people into patients. They can lead to an explosion of overdiagnosis and, in turn, an explosion of treatment. Even if a few end up being helped, labeling large numbers of people as abnormal and thus needing treatment is not something to be taken lightly. Small harms from therapy become magnified simply because so many are exposed them. Some, like Lara, get entangled in a cascade of diagnosis and treatment. And we all have to wonder about the paradox of promoting health by encouraging policies that lead more people to view themselves as sick.

Unfortunately, there is no scientific method or mathematical equation that will result in a single answer to the question of what should be defined as normal. But the practical reality is that the medical community is engaged in a relentless drive to narrow that definition. The process is most evident and most dramatic when we doctors change the rules. But there is also a more insidious side to the process—when advances in technologies change the rules for us.

# We Are Able to See More

*How Scans Give You Gallstones, Damaged Knee Cartilage,
Bulging Discs, Abdominal Aortic Aneurysms, and Blood Clots*

THE DISTINCTION BETWEEN ABNORMAL AND normal can be quite arbitrary, often hinging on the medical profession's choice of a single number. If your fasting blood sugar is 126, you have diabetes; if it's 125, you don't. But many of our diagnoses are based not on numbers but on what we can see. In the past, that meant what we could see with the naked eye; now what we can see has been dramatically enhanced by various imaging modalities: X-rays, ultrasounds, CT scans, MRI scans, and PET scans. Frankly, these are amazing technologies. Using radiation, sound waves, magnetic fields, and electrical energy, they can display anatomic structures in fine detail. Powerful computers digitize the information, allowing 3-D reconstructions of the images to be created that can then be enlarged and rotated in space. They enable physicians to precisely measure the dimensions of anatomic structures, the metabolic activity of tissue, and the dynamics of blood flow. And the resolution of these imaging technologies only increases with each passing year.

Imaging technologies are very helpful in finding the abnormalities that are making patients sick. But they are also increasingly able to find abnormalities in people who are well. Different mechanism than in the previous chapter, same problem. With the abnormalities defined by numbers, doctors are changing the rules. With the abnormalities defined by the medical profession's capability to see, the technologies are changing the rules. But the end result is the same: more diagnoses and more patients. While some may be helped, others are overdiagnosed—a patient is told he has an abnormality, but the abnormality is not destined to progress to cause symptoms or death.

### Seeing too much

During my last year of medical school, I had the opportunity to work in both technologically advanced academic medical centers (in San Francisco and Boston) and technologically deprived rural hospitals (in Alaska and Zambia). It was a formative experience for me. Bouncing from the medical center at the University of California at San Francisco and Massachusetts General

Hospital, both of which were on *U.S. News & World Report*'s list of best hospitals, to the Alaska Area Native Health Service and then an Anglican mission hospital in Katete, Zambia, taught me just how differently medicine is practiced in different settings—based in part on what is possible. But it wasn't apparent to me that the technologically intensive settings were always better. Don't get me wrong; there were times when access to imaging technology clearly improved patient care, but it was equally clear that there were times when it simply caused confusion, slowed treatment, and led to worse care. Yet even the technologically deprived environments had some imaging technology—X-ray machines are just about everywhere—and I also learned that sometimes even a simple X-ray can see too much.

After medical school I completed a rotating internship in pediatrics, surgery, obstetrics, and internal medicine before entering the U.S. Public Health Service as a general medical officer in Bethel, Alaska, on the Bering Sea coast. After two years in Alaska, I served at a number of other Public Health Service sites in the Lower 48. One was a small three-doctor clinic on the Warm Springs Reservation in central Oregon. It was mostly meat-and-potatoes primary care: hypertension, back pain, minor wounds, sexually transmitted diseases, and, of course, colds. In addition to the typical sore throats, coughs, and runny noses, many patients complained of sinus pain, for which we routinely ordered X-rays of the facial sinuses. I was struck (honestly, frustrated) by the fact that virtually every sinus film came back from the radiologist with a reading of sinusitis—a sinus infection. Did everyone complaining of sinus pain really have sinusitis? I asked my clinic director if he would entertain a small experiment—could I order a sinus film of myself? He told me to go ahead.

To order a film, doctors had to fill out a request slip outlining what they wanted examined and why. I felt fine, but in the "specific reason for request" box I wrote what I would have written for a typical patient in this situation: *thirty-three-year-old with sinus pain.* (I also checked the box saying that I was not pregnant.) The X-ray itself was quick, easy, and painless. I got the interpretation back from the radiologist six days later (films had to be hand-delivered to the hospital where he worked some fifty miles away; he had to examine them, have his interpretation transcribed, and then send them back). He wrote that there was an *ovoid density involving the inferior margin of the left maxillary sinus.* His conclusion? *This may well represent a polyp secondary to chronic maxillary sinusitis.* If you are not sure what that means, don't worry—neither was I. But it didn't sound good.

That was over twenty years ago. I have never had any sinus problems, then or now. If I really have a polyp, it has never once bothered me. It sounds like I was overdiagnosed, and all on the basis of a simple X-ray.

The finding that I had sinusitis was totally unexpected—I had no symptoms; the abnormality was a complete surprise. Surprise findings, as you might imagine, are often cases of overdiagnosis. But when people have symptoms, although the abnormalities discovered by our diagnostic technologies may not be a complete surprise, they can still be ambiguous. The abnormalities might explain the symptoms, or they might not. That's what frustrated me in the Warm Springs clinic. All of my patients with common-cold symptoms seemed to have abnormal sinus films. But was sinusitis really the explanation for their symptoms?

The classic symptoms of sinusitis have a lot of overlap with those of the common cold: runny nose, sneezing, coughing, and headache. When I worked at the Warm Springs clinic, the diagnosis of sinusitis was made based on some combination of symptoms and the findings of conventional X-rays. Now we use CT scans. CT scans are able to detect a lot of sinus abnormalities. Because of the overlap in the symptoms, one study using CT scans examined people with common colds to see whether they also had sinusitis. The researchers recruited thirty-one young adults with an advertisement seeking "volunteers with a fresh common cold."[1] Each volunteer had had his cold symptoms for fewer than four days, and each agreed to a CT scan of the sinuses. The results were staggering: 87 percent (twenty-seven of the thirty-one volunteers) had visible sinus inflammation on their CT scans. In other words, if we look hard enough, virtually everybody with a common cold also has sinusitis.

But most doctors would say that sinusitis and the common cold are two distinct diagnoses. We would say that colds are much more common and less concerning than sinusitis and that most people with colds do not have sinusitis. And we certainly treat them as distinct diagnoses: sinus infections are typically treated with antibiotics; common colds are not. But a CT scan makes the situation more ambiguous. Using this diagnostic technology, it appears that most people with a cold could also be diagnosed with sinusitis. But that would be overdiagnosis—virtually all of the volunteers were back to normal within two weeks, and none had been given antibiotics.

Although few doctors order CT scans for common colds, we are doing a lot of sinus CT scans for chronic nasal complaints. More and more, ear, nose, and throat doctors have specialized sinus CT scan machines right in their offices (just try Googling *office sinus CT*). If a simple X-ray can find chronic sinusitis in people who are not even sick (like me), imagine what a sinus CT scan will find in people with vague symptoms. Not surprisingly, scanning leads to far more chronic sinusitis diagnoses.

### The cycle of seeing more, finding more, and doing more

Sinusitis is just one example of a more general problem. Our diagnostic technologies are of such high resolution that we are discovering more ambiguous and surprise abnormalities. Both can lead to a cycle of more follow-up testing—including more scanning—revealing ever more ambiguous and surprise findings. And the bottom line is that more findings translates to more treatment—despite the fact that a lot of them represent overdiagnosis.

To initiate the cycle of seeing more, finding more, and doing more, two prerequisites must be met: (1) doctors must be scanning more (or using higher-resolution scans), and (2) there must be a reservoir of abnormalities for the scans to find.

### More scanning

There is no question that we are scanning more and that the resolution of these scans increases every year. (Some might substitute the word *improves* for *increases,* but I'll defer that judgment to you.) It is actually remarkably difficult to know exactly how much diagnostic technology is used because no single entity keeps track of it (which is because no single entity pays for it). Instead, diagnostic tests are paid for by many different insurance companies, federal and state governments, and by patients themselves.[2]

Investigators using marketing surveys have estimated that the number of CT scans done in the United States has increased from about three million in 1980 (when CT scanners were still fairly rare) to more than sixty-two million in 2006.[3] If accurate, this would suggest that on average about one in five Americans has a CT scan each year (of course, some people have more than one).

The most reliable data come from the Medicare program because it tracks (and pays for) the scans of virtually all Americans age sixty-five and older. And the increased use of CT scans and MRIs continued long after the technologies were introduced.[4] Since the early 1990s, per capita use of head CT scans has doubled. Abdominal CT scans have tripled, and chest CT scans have increased fivefold. While they're still ordered less often than CTs, MRI scans are increasing even faster: brain MRIs have gone up fourfold over the same time span, spine MRIs have gone up sixfold, and hip and knee MRIs are up more than tenfold.

There's no doubt about it. We are scanning more and more.

*A vast reservoir of abnormalities*

If we are finding more abnormalities, it's not simply because we are scanning more. There must be a reservoir of abnormalities in the population for these tests to find—abnormalities that we would otherwise never have known about.

To determine the depths of this reservoir, investigators have systematically scanned healthy people just to see what they find. They have examined asymptomatic volunteers looking for gallstones, damaged knee cartilage, and bulging discs in the back. Here's a quick summary of what they have found:

- *Gallstones*—In people without any symptoms of gallbladder disease (pain, nausea, or problems with fatty foods, for example), about 10 percent have gallstones when scanned by ultrasound.[5]
- *Damaged knee cartilage*—In people without knee pain or a history of knee injury, about 40 percent have meniscal damage in their knees when scanned by MRI.[6]
- *Bulging discs in the back*—In people without any back pain, over 50 percent have bulging lumbar discs when scanned by MRI.[7]

Of course, this quick summary obscures some important details: these percentages are lower in the young and higher in the elderly (and in the case of gallstones, higher in young women than in young men). For example, only 2 percent of asymptomatic men under age forty will have gallstones detected by ultrasound, while 80 percent of asymptomatic men and women over age fifty will have bulging discs detected by MRI.

So even if you feel fine, these scans can find a lot wrong with you. But these abnormalities rarely go on to cause problems later. Advanced imaging technologies create a lot of potential for overdiagnosis—and a lot of potential for unnecessary gallbladder, knee, and back surgery.

But if you *do* have symptoms, the potential for overdiagnosis from scanning is still considerable. Imagine you have knee pain. You have an MRI that reveals damaged cartilage—a meniscal tear. Just as it may have been tempting to say sinusitis was the cause of the volunteers' sinus pain, it's very tempting to say the meniscal tear is the reason for your pain. But a lot of people without knee pain—40 percent, in fact—have meniscal tears. In other words, damaged cartilage often causes no symptoms. So your meniscal tear may be the cause of your symptoms, but it may very well not be, particularly because there are a lot of other causes of knee pain; arthritis, tendinitis, and muscle strain, to name a few. If the damaged cartilage is not the cause of your symptoms, then being given that diagnosis as the reason for your pain is over-diagnosis. You can see why overdiagnosis matters. If damaged cartilage is the cause of your pain, knee arthroscopic surgery could help, but if arthritis is the cause, that surgery clearly does not help and in fact can only do harm.[8]

So the existence of a vast reservoir of damaged cartilage in those *without* symptoms makes the finding of damaged cartilage in people *with* symptoms ambiguous. The damaged cartilage may be causing the symptom—but it may not.

Judging whether an abnormality is actually the cause of a symptom is a big challenge for doctors. In a recent issue of the *New England Journal of Medicine,* an orthopedist described how he approaches ambiguous findings on MRIs of the knee.[9] He explained that damaged cartilage was more likely to be the source of the pain (and the patient thus more likely to benefit from surgery) if the patient was younger, had had pain for a relatively short period of time (measured in months, not years), and could clearly connect the onset of pain to an injury. But he also acknowledged that these guidelines were oversimplifications, that there were numerous subtleties involved in determining the cause of any symptom, and that ultimately doctors must base their decisions on sound clinical judgment. The science of medicine is not straightforward. It is often not clear what we should do.

One last example of the vast reservoir of abnormalities surprised even me. The condition is stroke—something most of us think of as fairly dramatic and obvious when it occurs. But a recent study in which investigators performed brain MRIs on over two thousand people—none of whom had had a clinical diagnosis of stroke—casts doubt on that assumption. The participants were members of the general population of Framingham, Massachusetts, who had been enrolled in the famous Framingham Heart Study. That ongoing investigation has long been considered one of the best-designed community-based studies; it observes people who are well, sees who develops cardiovascular disease, and thereby learns about risk factors.[10]

Incredibly, the MRI scans found that over 10 percent of these healthy participants had had strokes. The investigators called them silent strokes. As shown in figure 3.1, the probability of having a silent stroke is related to age. And what really struck me was the finding that 7 percent of those under age fifty had evidence of having had a stroke. That's really incredible. But whether or not we should be doing anything about silent strokes is a different question.

The reservoir of abnormalities in the general population goes well beyond gallstones, musculoskeletal findings, and strokes. A few years ago there was considerable enthusiasm for doing total-body CT scans. Some radiolo-

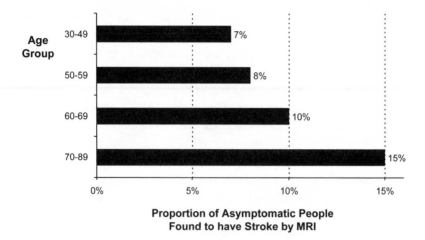

FIGURE 3.1 *Reservoir of Silent Strokes Found by MRI*

gists set up private for-profit clinics that offered detailed views of the insides of healthy people. One radiologist who had scanned more than ten thousand individuals noted, "The realities are, with this level of information, I have yet to see a normal patient."[11] He's about right. In a recent study of over a thousand people who elected to undergo total-body CT screening—people with no symptoms—86 percent had at least one abnormality detected. Because there were so many abnormalities found during the course of the study, more than three thousand abnormalities, the researchers calculated that the average individual had 2.8 abnormalities![12]

By revealing more and more abnormalities, imaging technologies shift the diagnostic spectrum of abnormalities by including increasingly subtle forms of abnormality. Thus, they also decrease the importance of the typical abnormal finding. In other words, because we can see more, the typical abnormality we see means less. Abnormalities that are detectable only by the new imaging technologies generally include less severe variants, those that are less likely to cause symptoms or death. The basic problem was well illustrated by an expert in fractal geometry who posed the deceptively simple question "How many islands surround Britain's coast?"[13] There is no single correct answer; it depends on how many you can see. The number of islands will increase with the resolution of the map used to identify them. But as the number of islands increases with improved resolution, and many previously undetected islands become apparent, the size of the average island decreases.

Check it out yourself. Get on Google Earth. And if you are not an Anglophile, try counting the number of lakes in Utah. When you view the entire United States, you'll see only one, and it's big—the Great Salt Lake. But then zoom in a bit. You'll find two more: Utah Lake next to Provo, and Bear Lake on the Idaho border near Wyoming. Now zoom in more. Multiple lakes will suddenly appear around the High Uintas, in the Wasatch Range, and on the Aquarius Plateau. But they are smaller. Zoom in more and you'll see more. But some will be less than a hundred feet across and only a few feet deep. That's not much of a lake; should it count? Eventually you'll have to deal with the question "What constitutes a lake?"[14]

And if you've got the time, repeat the exercise in Minnesota . . .

### Case study: Abdominal aortic aneurysms

Doctors being able to see more and more means that they will increasingly find abnormalities that mean less and less. The problem is clearly relevant to clinical medicine, particularly when the severity of a condition is defined by size. Abdominal aortic aneurysms are a classic example of this phenomenon.

The aorta is the largest blood vessel in the body, supplying blood to the head and arms, digestive tract, kidneys, and legs. It originates in the heart, travels upward in the chest, curves down into the abdomen, and finally ends when it branches into two vessels, one running to each leg. The portion of the vessel in the abdomen is called the abdominal aorta.

When a section of a blood vessel is stretched and weakened for some reason—high blood pressure, for example—a balloonlike bulge, or aneurysm, can form. If this balloon is in the abdominal aorta and it ruptures, it can cause a dramatic loss of blood and sudden death. The likelihood of that calamity is directly related to the size of the aneurysm. A large aneurysm has a high risk of rupture; a small aneurysm has a low risk of rupture. So while there is no question that doctors should treat large aneurysms, the benefit of treatment for smaller aneurysms is uncertain.

In the past, abdominal aortic aneurysms were found mainly by palpation—physicians used their hands to physically examine patients' abdomens. Under the best conditions, physicians can feel an aneurysm as small as five centimeters in diameter. There is variability in this method, of course: when physicians are directed to perform a physical exam to look for an aneurysm, they are far more likely to find it than when they are not specifically looking for it. The abnormality must be much more obvious to be detected during a routine exam. Today, however, most abdominal aortic aneurysms are discovered by ultrasound or CT, imaging that can show structures much smaller than three centimeters, which is the diameter of a normal aorta. A two-centimeter difference in what can be detected—less than an inch—may not sound like much, but it is.

A classic study of 201 men between ages sixty and seventy-five with hypertension and/or heart disease—the group most likely to have aneurysms—demonstrated just how much ultrasound can affect the apparent prevalence of aneurysms.[15] Five aneurysms were found in this population during physical examinations, while eighteen were detected by ultrasound. In other words, in the same group of men, ultrasound increased the apparent prevalence of abdominal aortic aneurysm more than threefold.

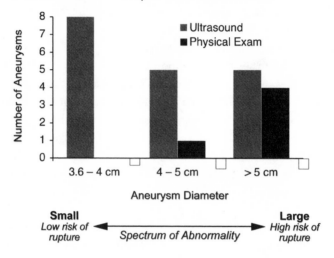

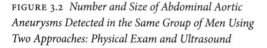

FIGURE 3.2  *Number and Size of Abdominal Aortic Aneurysms Detected in the Same Group of Men Using Two Approaches: Physical Exam and Ultrasound*

Figure 3.2 shows the results of the study. Most of the aneurysms detected by physical examination were relatively large and at high risk of rupture. Of course, ultrasound finds these aneurysms. But in addition, ultrasound detects many small aneurysms at low risk of rupture. Of the thirteen aneurysms detectable only by ultrasound, one was large (meaning greater than or equal to 5 centimeters), four were midsized (4 to 5 centimeters), and eight were small (3.6 to 4 centimeters). From the perspective of the clinician performing a physical exam, the prevalence of abdominal aortic aneurysms in this high-risk population of older men with hypertension is only 2.5 percent, and the most common type is greater than five centimeters. But from the perspective of the ultrasonographer, the prevalence of aneurysms in the same population is 9 percent, and the most common type is less than four centimeters.

The effect of ultrasound (and to a lesser extent CT) on both apparent prevalence and size of abdominal aortic aneurysms explains why the reported incidence of the condition increased sevenfold in the population served by the Mayo Clinic in Rochester, Minnesota, between 1950 and 1980, with the greatest increase—over tenfold—in the prevalence of smaller aneurysms.[16] About two hundred thousand Americans are diagnosed with abdominal aortic aneurysms each year, and almost all of the aneurysms—roughly 90 percent—are below the size for which surgery is recommended.[17] So when we use advanced imaging technologies more, we find more—but what we find are smaller abnormalities. The newly identified patients are at the lowest risk for having problems—and at the highest risk for overdiagnosis.

### *Switching from clinical diagnosis to scanning*

This principle is applicable well beyond diagnosing abdominal aortic aneurysms. The effect of moving from the clinical exam (a combination of information from the patient's story, symptoms, and physical exam) to diagnostic technology has been shown to be quite dramatic in a variety of studies. Consider the diagnosis of deep venous thrombosis, blood clots in the leg veins. These clots occur in people who are immobile for some reason, typically in the frail elderly but occasionally in the young who have been sitting for long periods (such as on a plane trip to Australia) or who have become bedridden by an injury.

Large blood clots produce swollen, painful legs. But people can have small clots that don't produce any pain or swelling. Studies of people injured in accidents—trauma patients—show that very few develop large clots and swollen, painful legs in clinical exams. But if the trauma patients are examined using duplex ultrasound scans, more than half of them are found to have clots, albeit small ones.[18] By adding clots found by ultrasound into the mix, the average clot has become a lot smaller and a lot less important.

The worst-case scenario for deep venous thrombosis is a pulmonary embolism—the clot breaks loose from a leg vein, travels toward the heart, and lodges in an artery in the lung. A blood clot lodged in the lung can have profound effects, making it difficult to get oxygen into the blood, creating a precipitous drop in blood pressure, and even causing death. (This is what happened to David Bloom, a young NBC correspondent embedded with the U.S. troops during the Iraq invasion who had been riding in a tank for many hours.) As you might imagine, the apparent prevalence of pulmonary embolism is affected by scanning. Relatively few patients with blood clots in their legs develop trouble breathing. Few are found to have pulmonary embolism by clinical exam. But with a ventilation-perfusion scanning, more than half of patients with blood clots in their legs are found to have small clots in their lungs.[19] Again, by adding the scan to the mix, the typical pulmonary embolism is now a lot smaller and a lot less important.

The advent of newer, higher-resolution scanning technology has further increased the apparent prevalence of pulmonary embolism. Ventilation-perfusion scans have been largely replaced by spiral CT scans. Spiral CT scans find a third more clots in the lungs of patients with leg blood clots than ventilation-perfusion scans do.[20] The effect of the increasing use of spiral CT is dramatic: in less than five years' time, the number of people in one state, Pennsylvania, diagnosed with pulmonary embolism increased 34 percent.[21] So the typical pulmonary embolism has gotten even smaller and even less important than it was five years ago.

Table 3.1 summarizes the numbers from these studies of aneurysms and blood clots.

TABLE 3.1 *Effect of Using Diagnostic Technology on the Apparent Prevalence of Various Abnormalities*

| Abnormality (Setting) | Prevalence of Abnormality Using | | Increase with Scanning Technology |
|---|---|---|---|
| | Clinical Exam | Scanning Technology | |
| Abdominal Aortic Aneurysm (201 high-risk men) | 2.5% | 9% (abdominal ultrasound) | 3.6-fold |
| Blood Clots in Leg (349 trauma patients) | 1% | 58% (duplex ultrasound) | 58-fold |
| Blood Clots in Lung (44 patients with clots in leg) | 16% | 52% (ventilation-perfusion scan) | 3.3-fold |
| | | 70% (spiral CT scan) | 4.4-fold |

So the principles that applied to diagnoses that were based on numerical rules (like hypertension and diabetes) apply equally well to the diagnoses that are based on what we doctors are able to see. Because smaller abnormalities are less likely to cause symptoms or death than larger ones, people with smaller abnormalities stand to benefit less from treatment. Furthermore, the number of people who have smaller abnormalities is far higher. It all combines to explain why smaller abnormalities are more likely to represent overdiagnosis.

Seeing more has created a lot of difficult judgment calls for doctors—sometimes it is really hard to know if detected abnormalities should be treated or whether it would have been better if they had been left undiscovered. The typical way we doctors get into this quagmire is when we order a scan to evaluate a symptom, not because we think the symptom suggests that an abnormality is likely, but because we can't imagine what else we can do. Call it a fishing expedition. And on fishing expeditions, seeing more can create real confusion. It's a setup for ambiguous findings—the discovery of abnormalities that may or may not be responsible for the symptoms—and overdiagnosis.

About a decade ago, when she was approaching eighty, my mother had a bad day. She had been her generally robust self (she was still hiking in the mountains of Colorado at the time) and I had never heard her complain about having a bad day before. She couldn't give me a very adequate description of what she meant (and I suspect she couldn't do any better for her doctor). She just couldn't remember the day very well. She said she was "washed out"—weak all over and not able to think very clearly. She denied having any more specific symptoms (chest pain, numbness, dizziness, fever, nausea, and so forth). She called her doctor and saw him a few days later when she was feeling better. He ordered an ultrasound of her carotid arteries—the arteries in the neck that supply the brain with blood. I'm sure he didn't really think she had had a stroke or even a mini stroke (a transient ischemic attack—the temporary condition that may herald a stroke). I suspect he was grasping at straws for common problems in the elderly and that he simply couldn't imagine what else to do. I can't fault him for this—I have also been guilty of ordering similarly illogical tests.[22]

The test came back abnormal—it showed a moderate blockage on one side of my mother's neck. I'm confident the finding was unrelated to her bad day. I say this because of both the duration of her symptoms (too long to represent a transient ischemic attack and too short to represent a completed stroke) and their character (nothing focal, just a general malaise). After she and I had a long discussion of the harms and benefits of performing surgery (which is a very difficult call in patients like my mother, those who have no strokelike symptoms),[23] she chose to do nothing.

That was over a decade ago; she has never had a stroke. But that diagnosis has stuck with her and has been raised a number of times by other doctors who have cared for her since. Some suggested getting it fixed; others recommended that she start taking medicines beyond aspirin; still others advised doing nothing—the course she chose. It was an ambiguous finding. And with the passage of time, we now know it was almost certainly overdiagnosis.

What happened to my mother happens all the time. Many asymptomatic people have abnormalities of some kind. A lot of people have episodes of vague abdominal pain. If we do ultrasounds in all of these people, we'll find a lot of gallstones. But most of the gallstones we'll find will have nothing to do with the abdominal pain. Lots of people have episodes of knee and back pain. If we do MRIs in all of these people, we'll find a lot of damaged cartilage and bulging discs. But most of the abnormalities we find will not be responsible for the knee and back pain. And a lot of people have bad days.

■   ■   ■

WHILE RELATIVELY FEW PEOPLE ARE said to have disease when doctors examine their outsides, relatively many are said to have disease when scanners examine their insides. The images from ultrasounds, CTs, MRIs, and the like are impressive. Doctors are able to see all sorts of abnormalities. The problem is that we see too much. Many people are now told they have abdominal aortic aneurysms, sinusitis, slipped or bulging discs, knee damage, strokes, or blood clots in their lungs and legs who never would have been diagnosed in the past. When we change the rules for conditions defined by numbers—like blood pressure—it's like rewriting our medical laws. When imaging technologies change the rules, the effect is more haphazard—different doctors have different test-ordering patterns, see different things in the test results, and make different recommendations based on what they see. Some patients are undoubtedly helped by these advances in imaging. But it comes at a cost—others are told they have abnormalities when those abnormalities are minor and not destined ever to progress to cause symptoms. These people cannot benefit from treatment; they can only be harmed. The problem is greatest when we systematically encourage the healthy to get screened to determine if they are in fact sick. And when doctors think about screening, it's typically in the context of cancer.

# CHAPTER 4

# We Look Harder for Prostate Cancer

*How Screening Made It Clear*
*That Overdiagnosis Exists in Cancer*

IT'S HARD TO IMAGINE THAT the phenomenon of overdiagnosis could apply to cancer. Physicians and the public have all been taught the basic facts about cancer. It's a horrible disease. It relentlessly spreads throughout the body. It invariably leads to death if not treated, and all too frequently even if it is treated. And the best way to treat it is to catch it early. So our goal as physicians is simple: find as many early cancers as possible. Until a few years ago, it was medical heresy to suggest anything else.

Then prostate cancer screening came along and forced us to alter our views. Suddenly it seemed that all we had to do was look for prostate cancer to find it. We found that so many men have prostate cancer—many more than we would ever expect to have symptoms or die from the disease—that we could no longer deny the existence of overdiagnosis even in cancer.

Cancer screening is about looking hard for cancer in those who are not sick. It is the systematic search for the disease in people who have no symptoms of it. (When we look for cancer in patients who have symptoms, that's diagnostic testing, not screening.) We are now looking really hard for cancer: testing more people, testing more often, and using tests that can see more. And the harder we look, the more cancer we find.

Of course, cancer is different than sinusitis or knee pain. The stakes are much higher with a disease that can kill you. But the treatment stakes are higher as well—cancer treatments can hurt and even kill you. You definitely would not want to receive cancer treatment if you didn't need it.

Like all the other efforts to diagnosis disease early, cancer screening is a double-edged sword. It can produce benefit: providing the opportunity to intervene early can reduce the number of deaths from cancer. It can produce harm: overdiagnosis and overtreatment. And it can do both at the same time. So while a strong case can be made for cancer screening, there are good reasons to approach it cautiously.

### A doctor becomes a patient

Isaac's not a patient of mine; he's a colleague. We are about the same age, in our mid-fifties. He is a fellow clinical epidemiologist on the faculty of a medical school in the southeastern United States. Over the past two decades, I've seen him at national meetings every few years. Isaac is an oncologist— a cancer doctor. He's got a certain intensity: he's bright, talkative, and very excited about his work. He investigates how pharmaceutical companies promote their treatments to oncologists. It's an important topic and it's his calling—he's highly motivated to do the right thing.

Last time I saw Isaac he told me he had been diagnosed with prostate cancer. Every year he had been testing himself by ordering his own PSA (prostate-specific antigen)—the blood test used to screen for prostate cancer. Although ordering tests on oneself may seem surprising, it's not that unusual for doctors to manage simple aspects of their own care. Isaac confided to me that he worried that his stature as an oncologist would be diminished in the eyes of patients if he had cancer, so he felt he had to make every effort to avoid getting cancer.

For a number of years his PSA had been below 2 ng/ml. That's good. The conventional rule of thumb had been to biopsy only those men whose PSA level was greater than 4. But in 2004, a study was published showing that some men with PSAs less than 4 nonetheless had prostate cancer. Some doctors began to argue that we should biopsy men whose PSA level was greater than 2.5. Others suggested that instead of basing the biopsy decision on the absolute level of PSA, we should biopsy men whose PSA rose substantially from one year to the next (the so-called PSA velocity). The next year, Isaac's PSA level went up about one point, to slightly over 2.5. He decided to get a biopsy.

A prostate biopsy for an elevated PSA is fundamentally different than other biopsies looking for cancer. Usually the trigger for a biopsy in other organs is a nodule (a lump of tissue) that doctors can feel or see with an imaging test. The purpose of the biopsy is to remove a piece of that nodule for pathological examination. Most prostate biopsies, however, are done because of an abnormal PSA, as in Isaac's case. In this setting, doctors typically can't feel anything or see anything by ultrasound. So there's no nodule to biopsy.

Because there is no obvious part of the prostate to biopsy, urologists generally take six to twelve separate samples to search for cancer throughout the prostate. Each biopsy involves removing a small core of prostate tissue with a fine needle. The urologists try to sample the prostate systematically, mapping the entire prostate gland into distinct regions and taking a biopsy from each. Isaac had ten needle biopsies. One showed cancer. That's all it takes. Isaac had prostate cancer. Whether a cancer is found in one of ten needle biopsies or in ten of ten needle biopsies, the patient ultimately gets the same diagnosis. But the latter case clearly represents a much larger, and likely more severe, form of prostate cancer than the former.

Isaac opted for the most aggressive treatment: a radical prostatectomy, total removal of his prostate. He didn't think it would be a big deal. But he was surprised. He said it was a big deal. He didn't feel like working for six weeks—he was wiped out from the surgery. And six months later he was still impotent. He said he and his wife were coming to terms with the loss of sexual activity, but it was difficult. Isaac questioned whether he'd made the right decision. He said to me, "You never would have done any of this, would you?"

I said no. That's because I don't get screened for prostate cancer and thus could never face this set of decisions (unless a doctor ordered one on me without my consent while performing other blood tests—something that happened to another colleague). But I may get prostate cancer and I may die from it. And it's possible that I would be a little less likely to die from prostate cancer if I got screened. We're not sure.

Did Isaac make the right decision to be screened? There's no way to judge. He may have made a good decision—he may have had a cancer that would have killed him if he waited until he developed symptoms, and now that cancer has been completely removed. Or he may have made a bad decision—he may have been diagnosed with a cancer that would never have bothered him if he had never looked for it. If that's the case, the only thing Isaac got from the diagnosis was the unnecessary anxiety of being told he had cancer, the unneeded surgery, and the subsequent side effects—like impotence.

Everyone knows the potential benefit of cancer screening: you may avoid death from cancer. Relatively few understand the more likely harm: you may be diagnosed and treated for a cancer that was never going to bother you. And, ironically, the fastest way to get prostate cancer is to be screened for it.

### How much prostate cancer is there?

A lot of men die from prostate cancer, an estimated twenty-nine thousand in the United States in 2008 alone. That makes it the second most common cause of cancer death in men (although it is dwarfed by the leading cause, lung cancer, which is responsible for ninety thousand deaths). The probability that a typical American male will die from the disease—the lifetime risk of death from prostate cancer—is 3 percent. Most men who die from prostate cancer are elderly; the median age of death is eighty.[1]

Even more men are diagnosed with prostate cancer than die from it, an estimated 186,000 in the United States in 2008. It is far and away the most common cancer diagnosis in males (excluding the non-melanoma skin cancers). The likelihood that a typical American male will be diagnosed with the disease—the lifetime risk of diagnosis of prostate cancer—is 16 percent. The median age at the time of diagnosis is sixty-eight.

And even more men have prostate cancer but don't know it. There is a reservoir of undetected prostate cancer. In the 1980s, pathologists at the Cleveland Clinic systematically examined seventy-two prostate glands that had been removed during operations for bladder cancer. There was no suspicion that any of the men had had prostate cancer. Yet the pathologists found that thirty-three of them, close to half, had prostate cancer. And among the men over age sixty, the findings were even more pronounced: more than half of them had unsuspected prostate cancer.[2] Some might worry that this study overestimates the size of the reservoir—that men with bladder cancer might be more likely to have prostate cancer than men in the general population. But there is little evidence that this is the case.

About a decade after the study at the Cleveland Clinic, pathologists in Detroit replicated this research and improved on it. They examined prostates from men who had died in accidents. The men weren't known to be sick or to have any cancer. And because they studied 525 men of different ages, the researchers were able to estimate the reservoir of prostate cancer in various groups.[3]

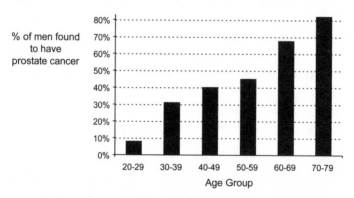

FIGURE 4.1 *Prostate Cancer Reservoir Found in Men after Accidental Death*

The results are striking. Remember, none of these men knew they had prostate cancer while they were alive. Even among young men in their twenties, almost 10 percent were found to have prostate cancer. And the proportion only increased with age. Among men in their seventies, more than three-quarters were found to have prostate cancer. That is a huge reservoir of prostate cancer. If over half of older men have prostate cancer but only 3 percent will ever die of it, the potential for overdiagnosis is enormous.[4] And when does this potential problem become a real problem? When doctors look harder in an effort to find small, early cancers.

### Look harder, find more prostate cancer

If there is a substantial reservoir of an abnormality, the more we look for it, the more we will find. Nowhere has this phenomenon been more clearly demonstrated than in biopsies for prostate cancer. Doctors almost never take just a single biopsy of the prostate. Because there is no obvious nodule to biopsy, the standard used to be six needle biopsies (a so-called sextant biopsy) to search for cancer in six different parts of the prostate. The decision to take six biopsies was totally arbitrary. It could have been four, it could have been eight, or it could have been virtually any other number. Nevertheless, the urologists used a systematic approach to try to sample the entire organ, performing three biopsies on each half of the gland at the top, mid-portion, and base.

But no matter how systematic the approach, it still boils down to extracting a number of samples, each about the size of a wood splinter, from an organ the size of a golf ball. Consider the numbers: six samples, each about twenty-five cubic millimeters, from an organ roughly fifty thousand cubic millimeters in size.[5] So the typical sextant biopsy specimens represent less than one half of 1 percent of the prostate gland. Some urologists reasonably wondered: What if we took more needle biopsies? Would we be able to find even more cancer?

Three separate studies addressing this question appear in figure 4.2,[6] each comparing six needle biopsies against eleven, twelve, or thirteen needle biopsies, respectively. In each case, the investigators found that the more needle biopsies they performed, the more prostate cancer they discovered.

There is one other needle biopsy study that warrants special consideration because the researchers looked so extraordinarily hard for prostate cancer. What was remarkable about this study was that their subjects were thirty-seven men who had previously been deemed cancer free not once, but on at least three separate occasions.[7] On each occasion, the man had had six negative needle biopsies. In other words, each man in this study had already had a total of eighteen or more negative needle biopsies. I would have thought that was enough. Nevertheless, when researchers performed what they called a saturation biopsy—thirty-two to thirty-eight additional needle biopsies—they found cancer in 14 percent of the men.

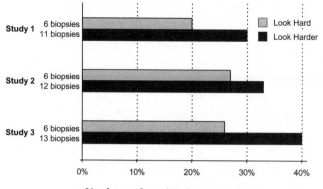

FIGURE 4.2  *How More Needle Biopsies (Looking Harder) Find More Prostate Cancer*

### Another way to look harder: redefine an abnormal PSA

Taking more needle biopsies is one way to look harder for prostate cancer. So is increasing the number of men who get biopsied by lowering the PSA cutoff that determines who is said to be abnormal. Just like the practice of taking six needle biopsies, the decision to use a PSA cutoff of greater than 4 as the threshold for biopsy was purely arbitrary. But it wasn't until a study was published in 2004 that we understood exactly how arbitrary it was. The prostate cancer prevalence study measured PSA in about ten thousand healthy volunteers, older men with no evidence of prostate cancer, and then biopsied *all of them,* regardless of their PSA. What they discovered was astounding: prostate cancer could be found at every PSA level.

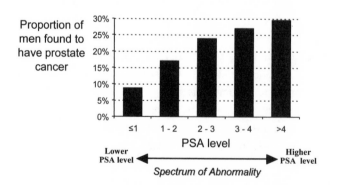

FIGURE 4.3  *The Proportion of Men Found to Have Prostate Cancer at Various PSA Levels* [8]

To be sure, the researchers were more likely to find prostate cancer in men whose PSA was greater than 4—almost 30 percent of this group had the disease. But they were able to find almost as much prostate cancer at a lower PSA level—27 percent of the men with a PSA level between 3 and 4 had cancer. Prostate cancer was even detectable in men with PSAs between 2 and 3, and, surprisingly, between 1 and 2. Even in those men with PSAs less than 1, 9 percent were found to have prostate cancer on biopsy.

While higher levels of PSA predicted more prostate cancer, there was no level that predicted no prostate cancer. So there is no obvious threshold for biopsy. Nevertheless, one of the major proponents of PSA screening looked at these data and argued that the new threshold for biopsy ought to be a PSA greater than 2.5.

Don't ask me where the 2.5 came from. It was another purely arbitrary decision. But I can tell you it was a decision that led Isaac to be biopsied and then diagnosed with prostate cancer. A lower PSA threshold means that many more men will be biopsied, and many of them will be diagnosed with prostate cancer.

The publication of the prostate cancer prevalence study and the new recommendation for a PSA cutoff of 2.5 led to my first invitation to appear on NBC's *Today* show. I was cast as the PSA detractor; William Catalona, MD, was the PSA advocate. Dr. Catalona was one of the early proponents of PSA screening, and although he didn't discover the test, he had been dubbed the "father of PSA screening." He was about fifteen years my senior and was a perfect gentleman both on and off camera. But he felt strongly that all men should be screened with PSA after age forty and that biopsies should be performed at what most doctors would consider a very low threshold (including below 2.5, if it is rising). I argued that his approach would expose thousands of men to overdiagnosis (in truth, millions) and would lead many to become impotent and have difficulties with urination; some would die from the surgery. I argued that we needed to tell men both sides of the story and let them decide. The interviewer was Matt Lauer, who did an excellent job guiding both of us to articulate our arguments in the five or so minutes we had on camera.

Off camera was a different story. Mr. Lauer immediately sought Dr. Catalona's advice on when and how he should be screened. This suggests two things to me: (1) that it is possible for a good reporter to balance both sides of a story even when he or she has a specific take on the topic, and (2) the paradigm of early detection is very persuasive.

To fully understand this issue, you need to grapple with the number of men potentially affected. Figure 4.4 estimates the number of American men sixty to sixty-nine years old, the age of most of the men in the prostate cancer prevalence study, who will be diagnosed with prostate cancer at various PSA thresholds. The data on the distribution of PSA level in the general population come from my own work and that of my coauthors. By altering the PSA cutoff, the number of men expected to be diagnosed with prostate cancer based on the findings of the prostate cancer prevalence study increases dramatically. For example, using the standard rule defining a PSA greater than 4 as abnormal, 5 percent of the population of men age sixty to sixty-nine will require a biopsy; about 650,000 men in total.[9] We know that roughly 30 percent of men with a PSA greater than 4 will be found to have prostate cancer on biopsy, translating to about 200,000 American men diagnosed with prostate cancer. If we change the rule and define a PSA greater than 3 as abnormal, then 13 percent of this population will be abnormal, translating to about 400,000 men diagnosed with prostate cancer. And if we change the rule and define a PSA greater than 2.5 as abnormal, that will translate to about 500,000 men diagnosed with prostate cancer.

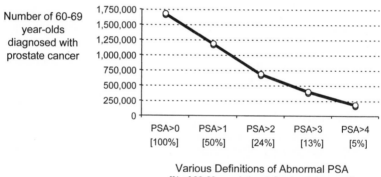

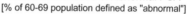

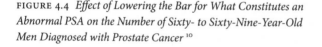

FIGURE 4.4  *Effect of Lowering the Bar for What Constitutes an Abnormal PSA on the Number of Sixty- to Sixty-Nine-Year-Old Men Diagnosed with Prostate Cancer* [10]

You can see the pattern clearly—and the problem. And where does it stop? If the goal is simply to find more prostate cancer, we might as well look really hard. Forget the PSA. Skip the needle biopsies. We should simply remove the entire prostate gland in every man and let the pathologists search each one for cancer. Of course, that's totally crazy. It would mean accepting all the complications of surgery. Millions of men would be harmed, and some would die, just to look for cancer. Yet this is the strategy that would find the most cancer.

### The heterogeneity of cancer progression

But should our goal really be to find as much cancer as possible? Imagine that we had a free, safe, and painless way to find cancers. Wouldn't we want to use it to find and treat as much cancer as early as possible? We now know the answer is no. It used to be assumed that all cancers relentlessly progressed. If they weren't treated, they would invariably grow, metastasize, and ultimately lead to death. But we are learning that this assumption is wrong.

We are in the midst of a paradigm shift in how we think about cancer. Our efforts to find cancer early with screening tests has shown that what pathologists call cancer encompasses a set of cellular abnormalities with very heterogeneous growth rates that vary from very fast to completely static. That's right, some cancers don't progress at all. Some cancers will never make a difference to patients. The idea that some cancers don't matter is a radical one for the medical field. It's as startling to us as the concept that humans were descended from animals was to nineteenth-century biologists, or the idea that continents plow through oceans was to early-twentieth-century geologists. These once radical ideas took years to become widely accepted and had to await the discovery of their underlying mechanisms (natural selection and plate tectonics, respectively).

Although the concept of nonprogressive cancers might seem implausible, scientists have begun to uncover biologic mechanisms that halt the progression of cancer.[11] Some cancers outgrow their blood supply and are starved; others are recognized by the host's immune system and successfully contained; and some are not that aggressive in the first place. These observations are leading to a fundamental shift in cancer biology.

Figure 4.5 is a simplified illustration of one way to think about the heterogeneity of cancer progression. It uses four arrows that represent four kinds of cancer categorized by their rates of growth. Each arrow starts at the same place: when the cancer first begins to grow as an abnormal cell.

Fast-growing cancers quickly lead to symptoms and death. These are the worst forms of cancer. Unfortunately, because the cancers grow so fast and because we don't screen people every day, they are often missed by screening, as they can appear in the interval between tests. Slow-growing cancers lead to symptoms and death but only after many years. These are the cancers for which screening will arguably have the greatest beneficial impact. This degree of heterogeneity in cancer growth—fast- and slow-growing cancers—has been understood for many years, in large part because of its implications for cancer screening. Cancer screening is the effort to detect the disease during its preclinical phase, the time period that begins with the formation of an abnormal cell and ends when the patient notices symptoms. Screening

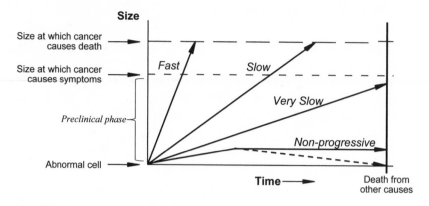

●    FIGURE 4.5  *The Heterogeneity of Cancer Progression*

tends to detect many more of the slow-growing cancers, because they can be caught over a long period of time; the tests find far fewer of the aggressive, fast-growing cancers, the very cancers we would most like to catch, because they are detectable for only a short period of time before symptoms appear.

Some cancers never cause problems because they grow very slowly. More precisely, they grow at a slow enough pace that individuals die of something else before the cancer gets big enough to produce symptoms. Dying before a cancer has time to cause symptoms is especially likely to happen in people with less time to live (because they are very old, for example, or because they have other life-threatening medical problems). Prostate cancer in older men is the most obvious example.

Nonprogressive cancer never causes problems because it is not growing at all. There are cellular abnormalities that meet the pathologic definition of *cancer* (that is, they look like cancer under the microscope) but they never grow to cause symptoms. Alternatively, they may grow and then regress—a pattern represented in the graph by the dashed arrow going down.

Overdiagnosis occurs when nonprogressive cancers and very slow-growing cancers are detected. These two forms of cancer are collectively referred to as *pseudodisease*—literally, "false disease." Since the word *disease* implies something that makes, or will make, a person ill, *pseudodisease* is an appropriate word for describing these abnormalities. These cancers are not going to cause symptoms or death.

The problem with cancer screening is that it cannot distinguish among these four kinds of cancer. So we can't tell who is overdiagnosed. While many hope that genetic testing of the cancer will help identify which ones are destined to cause symptoms or death, the field is in its infancy and it will take years to know how well it works. So for now, the only way to be certain that an individual has been overdiagnosed is when that individual is never treated, never develops symptoms of cancer, and ultimately dies of something else. But since most people who are diagnosed are also treated, this rarely happens.

### Population evidence of prostate cancer overdiagnosis

While it is extremely difficult to know if overdiagnosis has occurred in an individual, it is relatively easy to know if it has occurred in a population. The way we infer that overdiagnosis has occurred is by comparing the rates of cancer diagnosis and cancer death over time. Two distinct patterns of rapid rises in the rate of diagnosis are shown in figure 4.6—one is highly suggestive of overdiagnosis; the other is not.

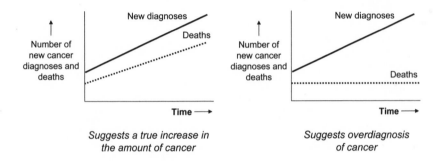

FIGURE 4.6  *Two Distinct Patterns of Rapid Rises in the Rate of Diagnosis*

In the graph on the left in figure 4.6, the rise in cancer diagnosis is accompanied by a rise in the feared outcome of cancer—death. This suggests that the new diagnoses are destined to be meaningful and that this is a true increase in the underlying amount of cancer that matters (as opposed to the very slow or nonprogressive cancers).[12]

In the graph on the right, the rise in cancer diagnosis is not accompanied by a rise in cancer death. This suggests that while there is more diagnosis, there is no change in the underlying amount of cancer that matters. It suggests overdiagnosis—the detection of very slow or nonprogressive cancers.

Some doctors will posit an alternative explanation for the right portion of the figure—namely, that there is a true increase in the underlying amount of cancer destined to affect patients but that improvements in diagnosis and treatment match the increase in new cases to leave the total number of cancer deaths unchanged. While possible, this explanation strains credulity. It is certainly not the most parsimonious explanation: it requires two conditions (true increase in cancer and improving medical care) instead of one (overdiagnosis). Moreover, it requires a heroic assumption: that the rate of diagnosis and treatment improvement *exactly matches* the increase in true disease burden. If treatment improvements outpaced the rise in cancer, mortality would fall. If the rise in cancer outpaced improvements in treatment, mortality would rise. For mortality to remain unchanged means that the rise in cancer exactly matches improvements in treatment. It's a stretch.

Now consider the rate of diagnosis and the rate of death for prostate cancer in American men. Figure 4.7 shows you these data over thirty years, from 1975 to 2005 (they are from the U.S. government's Surveillance Epidemiology and End Results program, better known as SEER, the nation's cancer registry[13]).

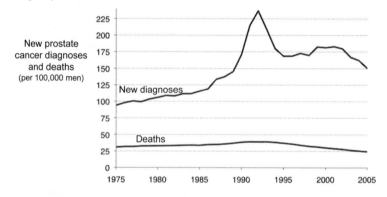

FIGURE 4.7  *New Diagnoses and Deaths from*
*Prostate Cancer in the United States: 1975–2005*

The top line, the rate of prostate cancer diagnosis, varies widely. The bottom line, the rate of death from prostate cancer, is relatively stable. In comparison, the top line looks more like a volatile stock market trend than a measure of the underlying amount of cancer in the population. In fact, I don't know of any cancer researcher who believes this curve reflects changes in the biology of prostate cancer. What it reflects is changes in medical practice, specifically in our practices regarding the diagnosis of prostate cancer.

From 1975 to 1986, the rate of diagnosis increased at about 2 percent per year, almost exactly mirroring the increased use of a urological operation called transurethral resection of the prostate, or TURP. The procedure was used to treat men who have trouble urinating because of an enlarged prostate (a disorder known as benign prostatic hypertrophy, or BPH). The operation involves shaving pieces of the prostate away from the urethra so urine can flow out more easily. As more men had the operation, more prostate samples were sent to pathologists to examine under the microscope, and more prostate cancer was found.

After 1986, the operation was performed less often because a number of medications that could treat BPH were developed. Consequently, the number of TURP-detected prostate cancers declined by about 50 percent between 1986 and 1993.[14] But the rate of prostate cancer diagnosis certainly didn't fall after 1986; it skyrocketed. From 1986 to 1992, as PSA screening was introduced, the rate of prostate cancer diagnosis almost doubled. As you can see, prostate cancer diagnosis really took off between 1990 and 1992, when the PSA test became widely disseminated.

After 1992, the rate did decline, as the reservoir of prostate cancer available to be found dried up and as more doctors became concerned about overdiagnosis, particularly in elderly men. But it has never returned to the level it was at prior to the introduction of PSA screening. Since 1975, there has been a tremendous amount of overdiagnosis. It's represented by the area under the curve in figure 4.8.

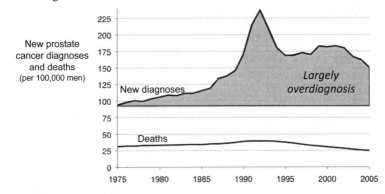

FIGURE 4.8  *Overdiagnosis of Prostate Cancer in the United States*

If all cancers detected early were cancers that mattered, the total number of individuals diagnosed with cancer over time would be unaffected by screening. Some individuals who were destined to develop severe cancer would simply be found to have cancer earlier by screening. Others who were not screened regularly would be diagnosed when their cancer progressed far enough to create symptoms. But the pool of patients with severe cancer would be relatively constant, and the total number of diagnoses would be stable.

But that's not what's happening with prostate cancer. There has been a lot of extra diagnosis, about two million additional men diagnosed with prostate cancer since 1975. And if you want to start with the rate of diagnosis in 1986, ignoring the effect of TURP completely, it is still about 1.3 million men.[15]

Without a doubt, all of these men have been made to suffer from the anxiety associated with a cancer diagnosis. But the bigger issue is all the extra treatment. Most have been treated with surgery or radiation. Surgery for prostate cancer (radical prostatectomy) has known harms: roughly 50 percent of men experience sexual dysfunction; a third have problems urinating; and a few, one to two out of a thousand, die in the hospital following surgery. Radiation can also lead to impotence and urinary problems (although somewhat less frequently), and it has a unique harm: radiation can damage the organ that sits immediately behind the prostate—the rectum. About 15 percent of men treated with radiation develop a "moderate or big problem" with defecation, generally pain or urgency.[16] While they cannot benefit at all, overdiagnosed patients can be grievously harmed by cancer treatments. It's not a small problem—over a million men have been overdiagnosed.

That's why the major federal advisory panel charged with evaluating screening services, the U.S. Preventive Services Task Force, has been so hesitant about prostate cancer screening. The task force is an independent panel of experts in primary care and prevention who review published studies in order to make recommendations about screening tests. They said that the evidence was insufficient for them to assess the balance of benefits and harms of prostate cancer screening for men under age seventy-five. But there was sufficient evidence for men age seventy-five and older. The evidence suggested that overdiagnosis was a huge problem; consequently, they recommended against screening.[17] In fact, the American Cancer Society recently revised its recommendations to reinforce this message. They said, "Because prostate cancer grows slowly, those men without symptoms of prostate cancer who do not have a 10-year life expectancy should not be offered testing since they are not likely to benefit."[18]

You may now have many questions about what happened to Isaac. What if he had had only six biopsies instead of ten? Would he not have been diagnosed with prostate cancer? What if he had followed the old rule and waited to have a biopsy until his PSA rose to greater than 4? Would his cancer have been just as treatable when diagnosed later? Or would his PSA never have gotten above 4 and he never would have been biopsied? No one has the answers to these questions. But there is an even bigger question you might raise: Should he have tested his PSA at all?

The fact is that at the time Isaac was biopsied, we didn't know whether anyone had been helped by PSA screening. Everybody was waiting for the results of two big randomized trials. In the spring of 2009, the two trials were published, one from the United States,[19] the other from Europe.[20] They represented an enormous research effort, almost twenty years of work involving over a quarter of a million men and many millions of dollars. Yet there is still some uncertainty as to whether screening saves any lives: the European study concluded that it did, while the U.S. study concluded that it did not. If anything, the U.S. data made one wonder if *less* screening saved lives. The European study found that screening *reduced* prostate cancer mortality by 20 percent. By statistical conventions, this is not a chance finding, but it is very close to being one. The U.S. study found that screening *increased* prostate cancer mortality by 13 percent. By statistical conventions, this is a chance finding. But there are some reasons to worry that screening could have the opposite effect of that intended.[21] So there's remaining uncertainty, despite two studies involving over a quarter of a million men.

That in itself tells you something: if there is any benefit from screening, it is undoubtedly small. In contrast, recall that VA researchers in the 1960s were able to convincingly demonstrate the benefit of treating very high blood pressure simply by studying about a hundred and fifty men over two years. Let's make the best-case assumption and suppose the European study is right. Its data give us some idea of the magnitude of the trade-off between lives saved by early screening and overdiagnosis in the best-case scenario: for every man who avoids a prostate cancer death, roughly fifty are overdiagnosed and treated needlessly. Some of my colleagues might argue that the actual number is closer to thirty; others might argue that it's closer to a hundred.[22]

Fortunately, in the United States the rate of death from prostate cancer has been falling—it's now down almost 30 percent since PSA screening started. But it's hard to know why it's falling. Unlike prostate cancer screening, prostate cancer treatment has clearly been demonstrated to reduce mortality in randomized trials.[23] Therefore, much of this decline must be due to improvements in treatment, not screening.

It is simply not possible to precisely quantify the benefits and harms of prostate cancer screening. Estimating the trade-off between a mortality benefit and overdiagnosis is problematic when there is uncertainty about whether the benefit exists at all. I believe there is some benefit; I know there is a lot of overdiagnosis. My best guess, given the data, is that for every man who benefits from screening by avoiding a prostate cancer death, somewhere between thirty and a hundred are harmed by overdiagnosis and treated needlessly. That does not strike me as a good gamble. But it doesn't matter what I think; it matters what you think.

■  ■  ■

PROSTATE CANCER SCREENING HAS BECOME the poster child for the problem of overdiagnosis in cancer. It is now clear that the amount of prostate cancer we find is directly related to how hard we look for it. If we biopsy more, we find more; if we lower the PSA threshold for biopsy, we find more. This is all possible for a simple reason: there is a huge reservoir of undetected prostate cancer. And these are not just theories. In the past two decades we have seen a dramatic rise in prostate cancer diagnosis. While there are tremendous debates about the effect of PSA screening on the rate of prostate cancer death, there is little debate about its effect on the rate of prostate cancer diagnosis. It has led literally over a million additional men to be diagnosed and treated for prostate cancer.

Our experience with prostate cancer screening has made one thing crystal clear: the goal of cancer screening cannot be simply to find more cancer. That's too easy. The real goal of cancer screening is much more nuanced: to find the right cancers, the cancers that matter. To be sure, overdiagnosis doesn't preclude the possibility that some men are helped. And there is likely to be a trade-off: we might be able to help a few men avoid prostate cancer death at the cost of overdiagnosing many others. So we need to balance the possible reduction in death against the chance of being diagnosed needlessly and put at risk for things like impotence, incontinence, and chronic diarrhea. Currently, from my perspective at least, we have lost that balance.

For what it's worth, Professor Ablin at the University of Arizona feels the same way. He recently published an op-ed in the *New York Times* entitled "The Great Prostate Mistake."[24] He wrote that "the test is hardly more effective than a coin toss" and "can't distinguish between the two types of prostate cancer—the one that will kill you and the one that won't." And why are his views particularly relevant? He discovered PSA. And he never dreamed his discovery would lead to such a "profit-driven public health disaster."

You might wonder if prostate cancer screening is a special case. In fact, it provides some insights about the problems posed by early detection in other cancers as well.

# CHAPTER 5

# We Look Harder for Other Cancers

IT'S TEMPTING TO BELIEVE THAT prostate cancer is a special case—the only cancer in which overdiagnosis is relevant.

To be sure, there are a lot of unique features about prostate cancer that make overdiagnosis a problem. First, we have looked really hard for prostate cancer, arguably too hard. Second, there is no other common cancer in which we are flying blind, forced to use the strategy of systematically biopsying all around the entire organ (rather than biopsying a specific abnormality we can see). Most important, more so than other common cancers, prostate cancer typically occurs in those at the highest risk to die from something else—older men—in whom a slowly growing cancer may not have time to cause problems.

So it's tempting to believe that prostate cancer is a special case. If you do, you're in good company, because I think a lot of doctors believe this is true. But you, and they, are wrong. Recent research suggests that some degree of overdiagnosis is probably the rule in cancer screening, not the exception.

But before I get to that, let me be very clear what I'm not saying. I'm not saying thyroid cancer, melanoma, breast cancer, and lung cancer can't be horrible diseases. Each one of these can quickly spread throughout the body—that is, metastasize—and lead to death. I'm not saying if you have early signs or symptoms of these cancers that you shouldn't go to your doctor. Quite the contrary: if you have an enlarging lump in your neck or breast, a mole that's getting bigger, or a new cough and some blood in your phlegm, you should see your doctor.

The question is whether your doctor should be looking for these cancers when you are well. While it may seem that screening can only help you, it can also hurt you: it can lead you to be overdiagnosed and treated needlessly.

### Lara's cascade

In chapter 2, I introduced you to Lara, a sixty-five-year-old New Yorker who got caught up in her doctors' enthusiasm to treat osteoporosis. As you will re-call, she was considered at risk for fractures and started on hormone replacement therapy, which was stopped following the publication of randomized trials showing it caused blood clots and breast cancer. She was then started on a bisphosphonate, which was stopped after she developed severe esophagitis. She was started on yet another medicine, which was stopped after she developed a painful rash. And then she was sent to an endocrinologist to figure out how to treat a disorder she didn't even have. Although he had no reason to worry about thyroid cancer, he carefully examined her thyroid.[1]

Remember that she was well. She had no symptoms of thyroid problems. She was screened. In this case, the screening test is just a physical exam to find lumps that may be cancer. Some doctors do this; some doctors don't. For whatever reason, Lara's endocrinologist did. He found that she had a lump in her neck. So do many of us. In one study, about 20 percent of normal individuals were found to have palpable thyroid nodules.[2] Lara's doctor sent her for an ultrasound, which confirmed that lump and detected two more. Most of us have thyroid nodules detectable by ultrasound. The same study cited above showed that two-thirds of normal individuals do. The doctor did a needle biopsy. And the biopsy showed that these lumps *might* be thyroid cancer. Often biopsies of the thyroid are equivocal (meaning neither definitely cancer nor definitely *not* cancer). The next step would be to remove some, or all, of the thyroid gland to determine whether or not the nodules were malignant. But a prudent surgeon put a stop to Lara's cascade.

### Thyroid cancer

He recognized that very few of us die from thyroid cancer. It's a cancer responsible for about 1,600 deaths annually in the United States. But the number diagnosed with thyroid cancer, 37,000, is more than twenty times that. There is a large discrepancy between the number of thyroid cancer deaths and the number of thyroid cancer diagnoses, even greater than the discrepancy between the number of prostate cancer deaths versus diagnoses (one to six). One possible explanation for this, as you will recall from similar issues with prostate cancer, is that we are really, really good at treating thyroid cancer. The other is less optimistic: that many of the diagnosed cancers didn't need treatment in the first place. And it doesn't have to be one or the other; both explanations can be partially right. You may wonder about a third possibility: that we are in the midst of an epidemic of lethal cancer. In this scenario, there are a lot of new patients developing cancer. They haven't yet exhibited symptoms or died from the disease, but they will. The conditions would have to be pretty extreme to lead to such a dramatic discrepancy; for example, a nuclear explosion could lead to a lot of new cases of cancer (in particular, leukemia) that might not show up in the death statistics for another few years. As you will soon see, this explanation doesn't pass the laugh test in thyroid cancer.

When it comes to thyroid cancer, I'm pretty confident that the major explanation is the second scenario. Many of the cancers don't require treatment. There's a tremendous amount of overdiagnosis of thyroid cancer. Just as in prostate cancer, there turns out to be a reservoir of undetected thyroid cancer in the general population. Pathologists in Finland systematically examined the thyroid glands in 101 consecutive autopsies of older patients who had died in the hospital, taking slices of thyroid tissue about every two millimeters (each slice was less than a tenth of an inch away from the previous one).[3] They found a lot of cancer. Over a third of the autopsied patients had thyroid cancer. And because many of the cancers were smaller than two millimeters, the width at which they took slices, they knew that they were missing some of them. Given the number of small cancers they did find and the number that they reasoned they had missed (which was a function of size[4]), the researchers concluded that virtually everybody would have some evidence of thyroid cancer if examined carefully enough. In fact, the researchers concluded that the smallest forms of thyroid cancer were so common that they should be regarded as normal findings.

We are just now beginning to tap this reservoir. Although few recommend screening for thyroid cancer (in fact, the U.S. Preventive Services Task Force—the independent experts who evaluate the nation's screening services—recommended *against* thyroid cancer screening in 1996[5]), doctors are apparently looking more often for lumps in the neck or stumbling onto them as an incidental finding of a CT scan, then ordering more ultrasounds of the neck (up fourfold in the past decade[6]), and doing more needle biopsies. The result is predictable, as shown in figure 5.1. Like all the national cancer data presented in this book, the numbers come from SEER, the National Cancer Institute's program to track cancer in the United States. The figure clearly shows that there has been a dramatic growth in the number of thyroid cancers found.

The death rate for thyroid cancer, however, is rock-solid stable. In fact, it is the most stable mortality rate among all the cancers reported in SEER.

This pattern should look familiar: it is the one that is highly suggestive of overdiagnosis. And there is further evidence that you can't see in the graph: most of the new diagnoses are small thyroid cancers, and all of them are papillary thyroid cancer, the least aggressive type.[7]

This is a simpler story than prostate cancer. In prostate cancer, the mortality rate has gone up a bit and then down a bit. The screening responsible

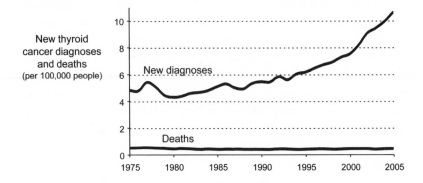

FIGURE 5.1 *New Diagnoses and Deaths from*
*Thyroid Cancer in the United States: 1975–2005*

for overdiagnosis in that case may also be responsible for some of the decline in the death rate. So, with prostate cancer, there's a potential upside to go with the downside. Here there is just a downside—a lot of overdiagnosis and no change in mortality. More people will be treated and have the thyroid gland surgically removed. The surgery can lead to harm. Most significant, there is the possibility of damaging the recurrent laryngeal nerve in the neck (leading to hoarseness, a weak voice, and trouble swallowing) or the parathyroid glands (disrupting calcium metabolism). Furthermore, everyone who has her thyroid gland removed needs to take medication for the rest of her life to replace what's been lost, namely, the ability to make thyroid hormone.

There is no discernible benefit.

### Melanoma
Most skin cancers are not melanoma. They are even identified in the negative: non-melanoma skin cancers. Non-melanoma skin cancers almost never metastasize and almost never cause death. Some doctors even wonder whether they should be called cancer at all. While they are far and away the most commonly occurring abnormality labeled *cancer,* non-melanoma skin cancers are not even recorded in national statistics (like SEER) because their health impact is relatively small.

Melanoma is the feared form of skin cancer. It does metastasize. It does kill people—about 8,400 deaths annually in the United States. But just like in thyroid cancer, far more people, about 116,000, are diagnosed with melanoma each year than die from it. And just like in thyroid cancer, when you see this large discrepancy you have to ask yourself: is this because treatment is so good or because many diagnosed melanomas don't need treatment in the first place? (Or did I miss another nuclear explosion?)

The reservoir of *potential* melanoma is large. I don't say this because of autopsy studies; you don't need to open up bodies to see the reservoir of potential melanoma. Instead, I say this based on a simple observation: a lot of us have skin moles. Some have more than others, but almost all of us have them. And while some moles are much more likely to be melanomas—for example, a big mole that's growing and has irregular borders and multiple colors—any mole could potentially be a melanoma. In fact, melanoma doesn't always arise from a skin mole. It may arise de novo. Adding to the complexity, melanoma sometimes appears in organs other than the skin (such as the eye and the intestine). And, as is sometimes the case with other cancers, there are people diagnosed with metastatic melanoma who have no visible primary site.

In recent years the public and primary care physicians have become much more aware of melanoma. You may have heard of Melanoma Mondays as a way to encourage people to have their skin checked. All of this combines to create a problem that is enormously frustrating for dermatologists. For them, there's no more important diagnosis to make than melanoma. Yet because almost all of us have moles that potentially could be melanoma, more and more patients end up in dermatologists' offices each year. This makes it increasingly difficult for them to serve patients with symptomatic skin conditions that aren't cancer. But dermatologists don't want to miss any potentially fatal melanomas. So they biopsy more.

A few years ago my coauthors and I studied the incidence of skin biopsies among Medicare beneficiaries.[8] We found that the rate of biopsy in this population increased 2.5-fold during the fifteen-year study period, from 1986 to 2001 (from 2,847 to 7,222 biopsies per 100,000). Predictably, over the same period the incidence of melanoma diagnoses in the same population increased at nearly the same rate: 2.4-fold. As we've looked harder for melanoma, we have found more. Figure 5.2 tells the story over the past thirty years for the United States as a whole.

As you can see, there is less an epidemic of melanoma than an epidemic of diagnosis. And again, there is further evidence for overdiagnosis that you can't see in this figure: most of the new diagnoses are small and very thin melanomas, those least likely to metastasize.

To their credit, dermatologists themselves have identified this problem. More than a decade ago some began to recognize that this growth was largely not an epidemic of melanoma.[9] But they are caught in a trap. All the forces— liability concerns, patients' concerns, financial incentives—line up to push

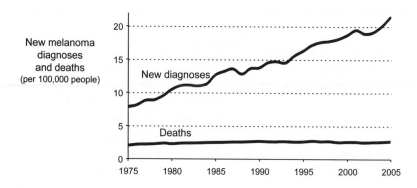

FIGURE 5.2  *New Diagnoses and Deaths from Melanoma in the United States: 1975–2005*

them to biopsy more. While there are substantial penalties for missing a diagnosis of melanoma, there is no corresponding penalty for overdiagnosis.

We certainly should not treat any patients needlessly. In cases of melanoma, however, I had always considered the treatment to be relatively minor. It's generally just a wide skin excision. This procedure has fewer harms than removing a thyroid gland, prostate, or breast. But a dermatologist I know took me to task when I made this argument. He pointed out that sometimes the surgery is more major, particularly on the face, and involves skin grafts and flaps. And he reminded me that the subsequent surveillance, looking for a second melanoma in patients who have already had one, makes some patients extremely anxious. And another time when I remarked that the problem of overdiagnosis had fewer consequences in melanoma, a young woman took me to task. She told me she had been diagnosed with melanoma and it had had an immediate and devastating effect—she was unable to get health insurance. A diagnosis of cancer is one of those preexisting conditions that make it very hard to find health insurance—a fact that the 2010 health-care-reform law will hopefully change. It was a potent reminder that simply being diagnosed with cancer can have real consequences, medical and otherwise.

### Lung cancer
From a public health perspective, lung cancer is the cancer that warrants the most attention. It's responsible for 162,000 deaths annually in the United States. That's more than breast cancer, prostate cancer, melanoma, thyroid cancer, and colon cancer combined. About 215,000 Americans get the diagnosis annually. That means most people diagnosed with lung cancer die from it. Our treatment of advanced forms of the disease is abysmal. If there was

ever a good candidate for screening, lung cancer is it. And it is really easy to identify a group of people at high risk—cigarette smokers.

But no major organization currently advocates lung cancer screening; some even recommend against it. The reason is simple. Three randomized trials completed in the 1990s showed that screening chest X-rays did not lead to a reduction in lung cancer deaths.[10] In fact, in two of the studies, screening appeared to cause *more* deaths. There was more lung cancer surgery in the screened groups, and lung cancer surgery itself can cause death.

The long-term follow-up of one of the studies—the Mayo Lung Study—demonstrated a persistent excess of lung cancer cases in the screened group.[11] Slightly over nine thousand smokers were enrolled: half were screened every four months (using chest X-rays and sputum cytology); half were not. At the end of the six-year screening phase, 143 lung cancers were detected in the screened group as compared with 87 in the control group—a difference of 56 cancers. Because this was a randomized trial, that difference must be a consequence of screening. But that's not enough to prove screening causes overdiagnosis; the difference could also be due to screening's advancing the time of diagnosis of cancers destined to cause symptoms (that is, the extra cancers diagnosed in the screened group during the first six years might have appeared in the control group in the seventh year, eighth year, or later).

In the subsequent five years during which both groups received similar care, the difference narrowed a bit—ten catch-up cancers appeared in the control group. These were cancers destined to appear clinically (typically with cough, bloody sputum, or a pneumonia) whose time of diagnosis had been advanced in the screened group. But extended follow-up over the next sixteen years identified no further catch-up cancers. Thus, the persistent excess of forty-six cancers reflected overdiagnosis. So even in lung cancer—what we typically think of as the most aggressive cancer—there can be overdiagnosis. After more than twenty years of follow-up, it appears that about half of screen-detected lung cancers found by chest X-rays and/or sputum cytology represented overdiagnosis.

Overdiagnosis is more dangerous in lung cancer than in most other cancers. From the Mayo Lung Study, it appears that almost all overdiagnosed patients had surgery. And the surgical treatment of lung cancer—removing a portion of the lung—carries a substantial risk of death (much more so than removing a thyroid, a piece of skin, or a breast). And the people who tend to get the surgery—smokers—also tend to be those who do least well with less lung tissue (because their lung function is already diminished by emphysema). In the Medicare data, about 5 percent of patients are dead within thirty days of lung cancer surgery. Nevertheless, there remains a lot of interest in lung cancer screening. Since we know chest X-rays don't work, the hope lies with a more recent technology: spiral CT scans.

CT scans, you will recall, see a lot. The same is true with spiral CT scans of the lungs. We now know that while spiral CT may find the lung cancers that kill people, it also finds a lot of other lung cancers. In fact, there is good reason to believe that it leads to even more overdiagnosis than chest X-rays.

Consider the numbers on smoker and never-smokers in table 5.1. The left half of the table shows you data from the classic 1956 article by Doll and Hill examining the mortality of some 34,000 male British physicians.[12] Sir Richard Doll and Sir Bradford Hill were arguably the two most prominent epidemiologists of the twentieth century. They played a major role in turning the study of what causes disease into a rigorous science. As you might expect, we can't use randomized trials to determine whether a potential harmful exposure actually causes disease (imagine trying to get a human-subjects review committee to approve a study that proposed to randomize subjects to either smoke or not smoke). Doll and Hill pioneered the observational study designs (cohort studies, case-control studies) we now use to investigate exposures we suspect are harmful.

In the 1950s one of the most pressing public health questions was: Why is lung cancer becoming so much more common? There were two competing explanations at the time: (1) the general decline in atmospheric quality (a few years earlier, London had had a killer smog, and midday in Pittsburgh could look like night); and (2) the widespread increase in cigarette smoking. Doll and Hill surveyed British physicians to determine which doctors had smoked cigarettes and which doctors had not. (Amazingly, from our current perspective, most of these physicians had smoked.) They measured the death rate from lung cancer in each group and established that it was seventeen times higher in smokers than in never-smokers. Of course, you knew that. (All right—maybe you didn't know the seventeen-times part.) And now you know that Doll and Hill are the reason you knew that.

The right half of the table shows you data from 2001 on spiral CT screening on more than five thousand volunteers, some of whom smoked, some of whom did not.[13] This study measured the rate of lung cancer diagnosis in smokers and nonsmokers. What it shows you is that with the advent of spiral CT, nonsmokers have about the same risk of lung cancer as smokers. It sure looks like the use of spiral CT has made cigarette smoking much better for you.

Of course, that's crazy. Doll and Hill's data from over fifty years ago are

TABLE 5.1 *Two Types of Lung Cancer:*
*One That Leads to Death, One Found by Spiral CT*

| | Death from Lung Cancer | | Spiral CT Diagnosis of Lung Cancer | |
|---|---|---|---|---|
| | **Death** (per 1,000 over 5 years) | **Ratio** Smokers to Never-smokers | **Diagnosis** (per 1,000 scans) | **Ratio** Smokers to Never-smokers |
| Smokers | 3.35 | | 11.5 | |
| Never-smokers | 0.2 | 17 | 10.5 | 1.1 |

equally relevant today—no matter how or where we study the issue, the finding is the same: smokers are ten to thirty times more likely to die from lung cancer than nonsmokers. This makes smoking the most powerful modifiable risk factor for cancers that kill people. Spiral CT technology is detecting a very different category of lung cancer, small abnormalities that meet the pathologic criteria for lung cancer yet are not destined to cause symptoms or death. Spiral CT is causing a substantial amount of overdiagnosis.

Looking hard for lung cancer can cause real problems. Just ask Brian Mulroney. He was Canada's prime minister for a decade (1984 to 1993). He was in the Conservative Party and was sometimes viewed as Canada's answer to Ronald Reagan. In 2005, he went to his doctors for a routine checkup. He was in good health. As part of the checkup, he had a spiral CT scan of his lungs. It showed two small but worrisome nodules. He had surgery to have them removed. Following surgery he developed pancreatitis, a rare but serious postoperative complication. He had to be moved into the intensive care unit. After a month and a half in the hospital he was discharged to convalesce at home. Then he had to be readmitted a month later to have an operation on a cyst that had developed around his pancreas—a complication of pancreatitis. He was in the hospital another month.[14] He didn't even have lung cancer—the biopsies were negative.

They were just checking.

But getting a checkup is not always the path to better health.

### Common cancers with little or no cancer overdiagnosis

Cancer overdiagnosis does not appear to be a major problem in either cervical or colon cancer. But that doesn't mean there is no overdiagnosis. There is overdiagnosis of precancerous abnormalities. That is part of what makes these cancers so distinctive: our focus is on removing precancer abnormalities rather than on trying to find early cancers.

## Cervical cancer

Cervical cancer was the first cancer for which widespread screening was initiated—the Pap smear was introduced in the 1940s. But the number of cervical cancer diagnoses didn't rise once the test became widely available; in fact, it has fallen dramatically since then (the rate of diagnosis is one-fifth of what it was in 1950).[15] That's good news.

Even better news: the death rate from cervical cancer has also fallen dramatically since then (the rate of death is one-fifth of what it was in 1950). And this pattern of declining diagnosis and declining mortality is continuing to occur. It is unambiguously good news. But I should share two caveats about cervical cancer screening.

First, while screening is widely viewed as the *cause* of decline in new diagnoses and death, the truth may be more nuanced. Other factors, such as improved hygiene and less sexually transmitted disease, may also play a prominent role. Factors other than early diagnosis can be extremely powerful: stomach cancer has experienced even greater declines in diagnoses and deaths, yet we have never screened for it. The explanation is a changing environment. (There is more to health than health care.)

Second, while screening is not associated with overdiagnosis of invasive cervical cancer, it would be incorrect to suggest that it hasn't been associated with any overdiagnosis (or overtreatment). It's just that the extra diagnoses are not labeled cancer. Instead they have been given precancer labels: dysplasia, carcinoma in situ, cervical intraepithelial neoplasia (CIN), squamous intraepithelial lesion (SIL), and, my personal favorite, atypical squamous cells of unknown significance (ASCUS). It's hard to know exactly how many women have gotten these precancer diagnoses, but given the rate of detection of these abnormalities, it's clearly a number in the millions. In fact, Australian researchers estimated that a typical fifteen-year-old girl undergoing regular Pap screening has a greater than 75 percent chance of needing a colposcopy—the follow-up investigation for one of these lesions—sometime in her lifetime.[16]

That's a lot of overdiagnosis of precancer for a cancer for which the lifetime risk of death is 0.2 percent (two per thousand). And it leads to a lot of treatment: cervical freezing, laser therapy, conization surgery (in which the core of the cervix is removed), and even hysterectomy (removing the entire cervix and uterus). Conization can cause fertility problems—and, of course, hysterectomy makes pregnancy impossible. In recognition of these harms, the American College of Obstetricians and Gynecologists recently issued new recommendations to cut back on screening younger women and to screen less often.[17]

*Colon cancer*

We've been screening people for colon cancer for at least two decades. Yet just as in cervical cancer, the number of colon cancer diagnoses hasn't risen—so again, there's no obvious evidence of cancer overdiagnosis. The number of new diagnoses has actually fallen since 1985, the time we began screening. That's also good news, particularly since the number of deaths from colon cancer is also falling. But the same two caveats apply.

I suspect screening is only part of the story. The number of new cases of colon cancer began to fall just as we began to screen. But instead of finding more cancers, we found fewer. For screening to explain the decline in the number of cancers, the mechanism would have to be the detection and removal of the precancer—polyps. But this argument fails because polyp removal did not become common until the 1990s, and there would have been a delay of some years between removing polyps and declining cancer rates. So the observed decline is a decade or so prior to what would have been expected as a consequence of screening.

So something even better must be happening. There's simply less colon cancer developing. Something about our environment (such as our diet) is better. That's great.

Second, while screening is not associated with overdiagnosis of invasive colon cancer, it would be incorrect to suggest that it hasn't been associated with any overdiagnosis (or overtreatment). The overdiagnosis that is relevant to colon cancer screening is the diagnosis of polyps. About one in three adults has polyps. This is far more than will ever develop colon cancer. Colon cancer screening does lead to a tremendous number of people having polyps removed. And once a person is found to have polyps, he or she is screened more frequently. That leads to even more polyps being removed. So many that the vast majority could not be destined to become cancer—instead, they could be considered overdiagnosis of precancer.

■　■　■

CANCER OVERDIAGNOSIS IS CLEARLY NOT limited to prostate cancer. It's a much more general problem associated with cancer screening. As we look harder and harder for cancer in the well, one of the unfortunate side effects is that we find more cancer than ever would have appeared otherwise. This, in turn, has led to a lot more cancer treatment. A urologist, Willet Whitmore, eloquently expressed the conundrum this way: "Is cure necessary in those in whom it may be possible? Is cure possible in those in whom it may be necessary?"[18] Another way of saying this is: Is cure needed in those who have cancers we can detect early? Is cure possible in those with the most aggressive cancers?

We now know that some people harbor small, innocuous cancers that will never progress to cause symptoms or death. The harder we look, the more likely we are to find these cancers.

The public should be aware that looking harder and harder for cancer is not the safest approach. And the doctors who recommend less aggressive screening (less often, starting later, or stopping at a certain age) or who are not as quick to biopsy might not be bad doctors; in fact, they might be quite good ones. The public should demand (and participate in) research that doesn't look as hard for cancer, doesn't find as much of it, but does find the ones that matter.

# CHAPTER 6

# We Look Harder for Breast Cancer

I THOUGHT I SHOULD SAVE breast cancer for last. It's undoubtedly the cancer that Americans have heard the most about, both because it is frequently in the news and because the color pink is so ubiquitous. Why has there been so much effort to make people aware of breast cancer? Mammography.

Before I go further, let me emphasize the distinction between diagnostic and screening mammography. A diagnostic mammogram is what we use to evaluate a woman who has a new breast lump—a diagnostic mammogram is useful in telling us what that lump is. This is the type of mammogram my wife had about a decade ago. She felt a new lump in her breast. She had a diagnostic mammogram. It was read as class 5—meaning the lump was almost certainly malignant. It turned out it was cancer and it had spread to a couple of lymph nodes. I was scared for my wife, worried about whether I could raise our ten-year old daughter alone. She had surgery, chemotherapy, and radiation. Fortunately, she is fine.

A screening mammogram is different—it's a test for women who have no reason to suspect anything is wrong. I want to be clear: the concerns raised here are about screening mammography, not diagnostic mammography.

There is no cancer for which screening has been more extensively studied than breast cancer. In fact, mammography screening arguably has received more scientific attention than any other form of screening. There have been ten randomized trials, each involving around ten years of follow-up. And these trials enrolled a remarkable number of women; over six hundred thousand have been randomized.

There is also no cancer for which discussions about screening have been more contentious. Mammography has been the subject of debate for decades. Several of my research colleagues have felt so discouraged by the level of discourse that they have decided to steer clear of the topic. Mammography certainly has a history of being the third rail of screening policy.

The juxtaposition of such a charged debate and such exhaustive scientific investigation should tell you something: there is a delicate balance between benefit and harm in mammography. Different women who are in exactly the same situations (that is, the same age and with the same risk factors for breast cancer) could reasonably make different decisions about whether or not to have a screening mammogram. It's a tough call. And one reason is overdiagnosis.

### *The never-ending debate*

The first randomized trial of mammography (and the only one ever performed in the United States) began in 1963. It was run by the Health Insurance Plan of Greater New York (HIP) in cooperation with the National Cancer Institute and is now known as the HIP study. About sixty-two thousand women were randomized. The intervention group in the HIP study received not only annual mammograms but also annual clinical breast exams (generally done by a surgeon). The control group received neither, and in fact were not even aware that they were in a study testing early breast cancer diagnosis. Unfortunately, this design meant that the HIP study could not isolate the effect of mammography alone; instead, it investigated the combined effects of mammography, clinical breast exams, and increasing women's awareness of the need for early treatment of breast cancer. (In the 1960s, this was potentially a very important element of the intervention.) After ten years of follow-up, the women in the intervention group who were age fifty and older were found to be 30 percent less likely to die from breast cancer. No reduction in death was found among women in their forties.

Based on the HIP findings, in 1973 the National Cancer Institute (NCI) and the American Cancer Society launched a nationwide mammography program. Despite the lack of evidence of benefit in younger women, all women age thirty-five older were encouraged to participate. Concerns were soon raised, however, about the radiation involved—both because the breast was known to be sensitive to radiation and because mammography then involved considerably more radiation than it does now. The concern was greatest for young women because they would be screened over the most years and thus be exposed to the highest cumulative radiation dose. In response to this concern, in 1976 the NCI and the American Cancer Society excluded women under fifty from the program.[1]

In 1988, both organizations revised their positions—now they advised women in their forties to get screened. They had been reassured that improved mammography hardware substantially reduced the radiation involved. Furthermore, the NCI had reanalyzed the HIP study and concluded that women in their forties actually did benefit from screening. But things did not stay settled for long. In 1992, the results of a large Canadian randomized trial were published.[2] The trial's design was similar to that of the HIP study—a reflection of the fact that its study director had been a HIP investigator. The intervention group received both mammography and clinical exams; the control group received neither. The difference was that this study focused exclusively on women ages forty to forty-nine. The result was surprising: screening did not reduce deaths from breast cancer.

By the end of 1992, nine of the ten randomized trials of mammography had been completed and reported in the medical literature. None of the studies (including the Canadian study) showed that mammography led to a reduction in death for younger women. Once again, some scientists concluded that screening should not begin before age fifty. Others were not convinced, however, pointing out that the limited number of younger women in the trials made it impossible to exclude a benefit. In February of 1993, the American Cancer Society reconfirmed its guidelines endorsing screening in younger women.

Three weeks later the National Cancer Institute convened an international workshop to summarize the trials.[3] The goal of the workshop was to assess the current knowledge and to identify issues requiring more research, not to make recommendations about mammography. The workshop concluded that the science showed a benefit in women fifty and older, but not in women in their forties. And the participants also recognized that mammography produced some harms: while they wrote about only the harm of false-positive results and unnecessary biopsies, one of my colleagues who was involved acknowledged that they also discussed the problem of overdiagnosis.

The controversy really heated up in 1997. In an attempt to resolve the uncertainty, the director of the NCI convened a thirteen-member panel of impartial medical experts and consumer advocates to review all the data and make consensus recommendations for American women. [4] This was a time-honored approach to difficult questions used by all the National Institutes of Health (of which the NCI was one); there had been over a hundred of these consensus panels in the past. The panel concluded that the data supporting mammography in women ages forty to fifty were weak. It wasn't clear that mammography saved any lives. It was clear that if it did save lives, it was only a few: less than one in a thousand women screened over a decade. The panel was more explicit about the harms: roughly a third of women would have at least one false-positive exam, and a substantial number would be told they had cancer (and be treated for cancer) when in fact they had been overdiagnosed. To them, mammography looked too close to call. That's why the panel members decided, for women in their forties, they could not make a recommendation either for or against mammography. They concluded instead that each woman should make her own choice.

This conclusion was greeted by outrage. One mammographer suggested the panel was condemning American women to death. Another called the report fraudulent, arguing, correctly, that nothing magical happens at age fifty. The director of the NCI said he was "shocked" by the outcome, leading many to wonder why he'd convened the panel if he already knew there was a right answer. The former head of the National Institutes of Health and a prominent supporter of women's health issues, Bernadine Healy, told a *New York Times* reporter that she was "very disturbed that a group of so-called experts challenged the notion of early detection," although she acknowledged she had not read the report.[5]

The politicians didn't behave much better. Senator Arlen Specter (R-PA) summoned the panel's chairman to defend the recommendation at a special hearing of the Senate Appropriations Subcommittee on Labor, Health and Human Services, and Related Agencies. The Senate went on to vote for a nonbinding resolution supporting mammography for women in their forties. No one wanted to be on the wrong side of this issue—the vote was 98 to 0. The director of the NCI, now under considerable political pressure, asked his advisory board to review the panel's recommendation. At first the board members declined, not wanting to interfere with the time-honored process, but eventually they voted 17 to 1 in favor of recommending mammography to all women in their forties.

Twelve years later, in 2009, a similar brouhaha erupted when the U.S. Preventive Services Task Force came to the conclusion that women should be screened for breast cancer starting at age fifty instead of forty.[6] The timing couldn't have been worse. Even though the members of the task force had been appointed by the Bush administration and had reached their conclusions a year earlier, the public announcement of their findings coincided with the Obama administration's efforts to reform health care. So now recommendations about mammography got confused with a much bigger issue: the control of health-care costs. Despite the fact that the members of the task force explicitly stated they had not considered costs in their recommendation, administration opponents characterized their findings as being the onset of rationing and a prelude to the brave new world of "death panels."

The secretary of health and human services, Kathleen Sebelius, quickly distanced the administration from the findings, and hearings were hastily scheduled in both the House and Senate to determine the future of the U.S. Preventive Services Task Force itself. Notably, there was support for the guidelines from leading women's-health groups: Breast Cancer Action, the National Breast Cancer Coalition, and the National Women's Health Network. But the mammography third rail was still hot. Many politicians, policy makers, and doctors apparently didn't want to touch it—they took the safe course and opposed the recommendation.

### Benefits and harms

To be sure, breast cancer is a very important cancer from a public health perspective and arguably the most important cancer for nonsmoking women to worry about; that's the cancer they are at the highest risk of dying from. (For smokers of either gender, lung cancer poses by far the greatest risk of cancer death.) Breast cancer kills about forty thousand women each year in the United States. So screening certainly deserves careful consideration. But every year, breast cancer is diagnosed in about a quarter of a million women—about six times as many as die from it. This isn't as dramatic a difference as in thyroid cancer or melanoma, but it should still lead you to wonder about the possibility of overdiagnosis.

To really understand the debate, you need to know the real benefits and harms of mammography. This is not as simple as it may sound: while mammography has real benefits, there are a number of common assumptions about the benefits that are simply not true. And while many people are aware of some obvious downsides of mammography, the most important harm is the least well known. My perception is that the benefits have been systematically exaggerated, and the harms have been minimized or, worse, not disclosed. And then there is the unfortunate reality that despite the tremendous effort and the tremendous number of women involved, the randomized trials did not provide definitive answers.

### The real benefit of mammography

Based on all the studies, the U.S. Preventive Services Task Force estimated that the benefit of mammography was about a 15 percent reduction in the chance of dying from breast cancer.[7] To acknowledge that some imprecision exists (and to be able to work with a nice round number), I'll use a more optimistic estimate: a 20 percent reduction. If all women were destined to die from breast cancer, this would represent a tremendous benefit—we would have to screen only five women to avoid one death. But of course, most women are not destined to die from breast cancer, so mammography cannot help them.

The situation is analogous to how the spectrum of abnormality relates to the benefit of treatment: people with milder abnormalities stand to benefit less from treatment than those with severe ones. In screening, you should think about the spectrum of risk: people at low risk for the particular disease stand to benefit less from screening than those at high risk. It's the reason that no one argues for mammography screening in men (although men do die from breast cancer, albeit rarely).

With the exception of a few relatively uncommon genetic mutations, by far the most important risk factor for breast cancer is a woman's age. Thus, the best way to consider the benefit of mammography is as a function of age, as shown in table 6.1.

TABLE 6.1  *Benefits of Mammography*[8]

| Age | Among 1,000 women screened for 10 years, the number who: | |
| | Benefit (avoid a breast cancer death) | Do not benefit |
| --- | --- | --- |
| 40 | 0.5 | 999.5 |
| 45 | 0.7 | 999.3 |
| 50 | 1.0 | 999.0 |
| 55 | 1.4 | 998.6 |
| 60 | 1.7 | 998.3 |
| 65 | 2.0 | 998.0 |
| 70 | 2.3 | 997.7 |

Two realities stand out from the table. First, most women will not benefit from mammography—for example, about two thousand forty-year-old women need to be screened over ten years for one woman to benefit. The reason is simple: most women are not destined to get breast cancer. Of the few who are, more than two-thirds can be equally well treated no matter how they're diagnosed.[9] Thus, even fewer are destined to die from breast cancer. And mammography will help avoid this outcome in only one in five of them.

There is a second reality highlighted in the table: while the benefit does rise with age, there's no obvious age to draw a line based on the magnitude of benefit; it rises steadily, but never dramatically. Some of this is an artifact of assuming that the magnitude of the death reduction is constant across age. There are some reasons to believe that mammography might be less effective in women in their forties: these women tend to have denser breasts (in which cancers are more difficult to detect) and the few young women who do develop breast cancer tend to have a fast-growing form of the disease (a form more likely to be missed by screening, as it appears in the interval between screening tests). But even if the number of women in their forties who benefit from mammography dropped a bit,[10] the decision about whether or not to have mammography is probably less about age and more about personal preference—how individuals value the trade-off of benefit and harms.

### Assumed—but not real—benefits of mammography

I am often asked about three assumed benefits of mammography: less metastatic disease, less need for aggressive treatments, and important reassurance. Unfortunately, reviewing the actual evidence suggests that these "benefits" are limited or nonexistent.

It is often assumed that in addition to reducing the risk of breast cancer death, mammography reduces the risk of developing of metastatic cancer; that is, cancer that has spread beyond the breast and reached other organs, such as the lungs, bones, brain, and liver. The randomized trials don't specifically address this question. Unfortunately, developing metastatic breast cancer and dying from breast cancer are fairly close to being the same outcome. In other words, most women with metastatic breast cancer ultimately die from breast cancer (about 90 percent in the SEER data). Thus most of the reduction in metastatic disease is already captured in the death benefit. But there may still be a little metastatic disease that could be prevented in women who ultimately die from other causes. The little extra benefit that could possibly exist is more than captured by my rounding up to a 20 percent reduction in mortality, rather than a 15 percent reduction. So you can think of table 6.1 as capturing the benefit of avoiding both breast cancer death and metastatic breast cancer.

It is also often assumed that mammography allows women to avoid more aggressive treatment. The idea is straightforward: mammography detects cancer before a woman develops a lump or other symptoms. Because these cancers are caught earlier, they are easier to treat. That should translate into fewer mastectomies. While this may be the case for selected individuals, the randomized trials show that mammography overall has had the opposite effect: it has led to more mastectomies, about 20 percent more, not fewer.[11] The reason is that mammography increases both the number of women diagnosed with invasive breast cancer and the number found to have multiple microscopic cancers distributed throughout the breast, for which mastectomy is recommended.

But far and away the most common question I get goes something like this: "Why aren't you talking more about the benefit of having a normal mammogram? It provides important reassurance value." To me, reassurance implies your being told that you don't have breast cancer now and you won't develop it in the near future. To be honest, I believe we have overstated how much reassurance a normal mammogram provides.

Ideally, a normal mammogram would be definitive. However, mammograms miss about one-quarter of cancers that are destined to appear during the following year.[12] There are two reasons why this happens: one is that the image (or the radiologist looking at the image) fails to detect a cancer that is there; the other is that the cancer wasn't there at the time of the test but started growing soon after. Unfortunately, the second explanation is a marker for a more deadly cancer, because it indicates a fast-growing cancer.[13] So a normal mammogram doesn't mean you won't get cancer in the next year, though it does mean you could reasonably expect that the risk is reduced by about three-quarters for that year, that is, until you get your next mammogram.

Does a normal mammogram provide much assurance beyond that period? Sadly, I'm afraid the answer is no. A normal mammogram this year has little predictive value for next year. The fact is that most mammogram-detected cancers are preceded by normal mammograms the previous year. Long-term follow-up of over 215,000 women who had had normal mammograms in New Mexico (one of the states that keep excellent cancer data and one of the original SEER registries) showed that their risk of developing cancer over the next seven years was almost exactly that of similar-age women in the general population.[14] So while a normal mammogram may provide some reassurance that you are less likely to be diagnosed with cancer before your next mammogram, it confers little information beyond that. If women are reassured about the long term, it is largely an illusion.

I wonder if a big part of the emotion captured in the word *reassurance* is actually relief—relief that you don't have cancer right now. Of course, the fear that you might have it may be due to the screening effort itself. There could be no relief unless there was a fear of breast cancer to begin with. I think that some—perhaps much—of the fear that women have about breast cancer is the result of the screening. One might imagine producing relief by making people take a test and telling them all that some will fail. Those that pass will feel relief. But one could avoid the need for relief by not promoting and giving the test in the first place. There has got to be some other reason for the test. The reason to undergo mammography is to avoid a breast cancer death. That is the benefit of a screening test.

*Harms of mammography*

Whether because they have the disease, know someone with the disease, or are worried that they may get the disease, a lot of people have breast cancer in their lives. While some of this reflects the prevalence of the disease, much of it reflects our use of mammography. To encourage women to get mammography screening, women had to be made more aware of the disease. The most effective strategy to do this is to scare them. In this country, women have been indoctrinated to believe that it is dangerous not to be screened; they're told to "take the test, not the chance." An old ad from the American Cancer Society even suggested that women were crazy if they forwent screening: "If a woman doesn't have a mammogram she needs more than her breasts examined." So, ironically, the first harmful side effect of mammography is that its promotion has led to a more anxious population.

Then there are the harms of the testing process itself. While many women find mammograms to be an acceptable test, many others find it more than uncomfortable; some find it quite painful. Then there's the problem that mammograms are too often read as abnormal. The issue is particularly large in this country, where it has been estimated that nearly half of women will have at least one film read as abnormal during a ten-year course of annual mammography.[15] Some women will have additional films recommended immediately; some will be told to wait for a repeat exam in six months; some will be scheduled for biopsy; and a few will get stuck in a seemingly endless cycle of testing because their mammograms are somehow concerning. All will worry that they might have breast cancer. But the vast majority don't have it.

This is the problem of false-positive results: the mammogram is positive (that is, read as abnormal), but no cancer is found—thus, the mammogram is falsely positive. Consider them to be false alarms. What little research that has been done on the topic suggests most women largely accept this harm. But while writing this I happened to interview a prospective employee who told me she had decided to stop getting mammograms precisely for this reason. She had had a worrisome mammogram, had gone through more testing, and ultimately had a painful (and disfiguring) open biopsy. She knew about the benefit, but she had also experienced one of the harms. She decided forgo both and to stop getting screening mammograms.

There is another harm to mammography that is less often mentioned: the harm of advancing the time of cancer diagnosis without any influence on long-term outcomes. A mammographically detected cancer can fall into one of three buckets: (1) a clinically important cancer that is more curable because it is caught early (that's the benefit of mammography); (2) an over-diagnosed cancer (which I'll get to in a minute); or (3) a clinically important cancer that is *not* more curable when caught early. Actually, most—over 90 percent, in fact—of mammographically detected cancers fall into one of the last two categories.[16] The patient in the final category may be cured of her disease regardless of whether it is detected clinically (after symptoms arise) or by screening, *or* she may be destined to die from her disease regardless of when and how it's caught. The effect of mammography in this category is straightforward: women are told they have breast cancer and are treated for breast cancer earlier than they would have been without mammography. They don't benefit from this early detection; instead, they are simply turned into breast cancer patients at a younger age.

The deputy director of the Canadian National Breast Cancer Study was grateful she avoided this harm. At age sixty-nine, she saw a surgeon to evaluate a discomfort in her breast. A diagnostic mammogram detected an obvious cancer, which was confirmed following surgery. It was an early cancer; there were no signs of spread. There was every reason to believe that she would do well. The surgeon examined her previous mammograms and, although it was smaller, the cancer was present. It hadn't been missed; she had had a six-month follow-up film at the time and it hadn't grown. What is remarkable is that these films were from nine years earlier. She could have become a patient at age sixty and had the same outcome; she was glad her diagnosis was delayed.[17]

### Mammography and overdiagnosis
Higher anxiety about breast cancer, false alarms, and turning people into patients at a younger age than necessary are all harms of screening mammography. But from an individual's perspective, at least, none is as important as the harm of overdiagnosis. And as you now know, the prerequisite for over-diagnosis is the existence of an undetected disease reservoir.

Based on seven autopsy studies involving more than a thousand women, somewhere between 2 and 40 percent of women who were not known to have breast cancer—and who died for some reason other than breast cancer—nonetheless had pathologic evidence of breast cancer upon examination.[18] To be sure, 2 to 40 percent is a fairly broad range. This variability has a number of explanations. Different studies have looked at different groups of women, particularly women of different ages. Like most cancers, breast cancer is more common in the elderly. Different studies involved different pathologists, who undoubtedly had different thresholds for calling an abnormality cancer (particularly a small abnormality). And finally, different studies used different degrees of scrutiny—some looked harder than others. At one extreme, investigators examined more than two hundred slices per breast; at the other, fewer than ten.

No matter how variable, however, these data show that some women have breast cancer but will never know it, unless, of course, we look hard for it. And now there is compelling evidence that mammography is beginning to find it.

Throughout Europe—including Denmark, Italy, Norway, Sweden, and the United Kingdom—the implementation of screening mammography in the 1980s and '90s was associated with a substantial increase in the number of breast cancers detected among women of screening age (in Europe, generally fifty and older).[19] These programs were all introduced by governments to populations that received government-funded health care. Thus, from a research perspective, they shared a very desirable feature: there was a fairly well-defined start date before which most women were not getting mammograms and after which most women were.

If there were no overdiagnosis, then the total number of individuals diagnosed with cancer would be unaffected by screening. A rise in the number of breast cancers following the initiation of screening is expected (some people do have cancers destined to appear later that can be detected by screening),[20] but if there is truly no overdiagnosis, that rise will be offset by reductions in the numbers of cancers detected later. In other words, if all cancers detected early through screening were ultimately going to be clinically evident (typically when a woman notices a new breast lump and then seeks medical care to evaluate it), one would expect a subsequent decline in the number of cancers detected clinically later in time. Since the cancers would have been detected and treated in women of screening age, the reduction should become evident as the women age and stop screening (in Europe, generally around ages sixty-five to seventy). Throughout Europe this reduction has largely failed to appear.

Figure 6.1 illustrates what I mean. The data are from the United Kingdom.[21] The dashed lines are trend lines—they reflect projected breast cancer incidence based on trends prior to the introduction of mammography. The lower solid line shows what actually happened to women ages fifty through sixty-four—the age group that was screened. Soon after screening was initiated, the incidence of breast cancer rose sharply. That was expected. What was unexpected was that the increase was sustained—now in the United

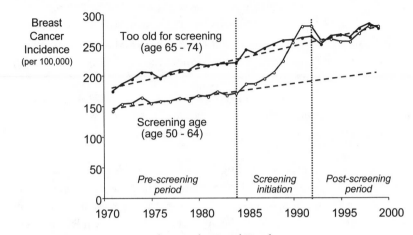

FIGURE 6.1  *Breast Cancer Incidence in the United Kingdom*

Kingdom, breast cancer incidence of women fifty through sixty-four is virtually the same as in women some ten years older who were not screened.

This rise in itself does not prove that overdiagnosis is occurring. It is still possible that mammography in this age group is simply advancing the time of diagnosis of cancers that would otherwise appear in the sixty-five to seventy-five age group. But if that is the case, incidence in the group that is too old for screening should fall. And as you can see, the incidence in women ages sixty-five to seventy-five has been unaffected by screening.

This is compelling evidence for overdiagnosis. It has many European screening experts worried. Clearly, some of the cancers found by mammography are not destined to progress to become clinically evident. A substantial portion even appear to regress.[22]

In the United States, the picture is murkier. We never started a national screening program, and even if we decided to, there's no single health-care system that can reach all eligible women at the same time. So in the United States, there was no obvious start date for breast cancer screening. Instead, mammography use trickled in during the 1970s and the 1980s. Figure 6.2 displays its impact on breast cancer detection determined by using the SEER data.

The little spike in 1974 has an interesting story. You may have noticed that this graph starts two years earlier than those in earlier chapters: in 1973 instead of 1975. In general, the SEER data reports begin with the year 1975, but the SEER program actually started in 1973. Because I knew that spike was there, I went back and requested the data for 1973 and 1974. The spike represents the Betty Ford effect.

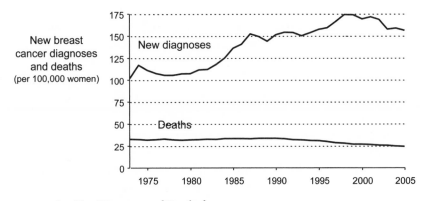

FIGURE 6.2  *New Diagnoses and Deaths from Breast Cancer in the United States, 1973–2005*

I learned about the Betty Ford effect as a student at the School of Public Health at the University of Washington. Betty Ford was diagnosed with breast cancer in 1974—a few weeks after her husband became president of the United States. (Ironically, two weeks later, the vice president's wife, Happy Rockefeller, was also diagnosed with breast cancer.) Mrs. Ford was very candid about her diagnosis. Prior to this, breast cancer was rarely mentioned openly. But hers was widely covered in the media. She was arguably the first high-profile public figure to share her breast cancer with the world and to make a public case for early detection.

The publicity surrounding her cancer gave a major boost to what had been lackluster recruiting for the breast-screening project sponsored by the National Cancer Institute and the American Cancer Society. In short, in 1974 a lot of women who had never gotten mammograms got them, and the number of cancers diagnosed increased sharply. The Betty Ford effect is a potent reminder that how much cancer we find is a reflection of how hard we look for it.

Now let's get to the bigger picture. As mammography was introduced during the 1970s and 1980s, the rate of breast cancer diagnoses increased about 50 percent. Some of this rise may have reflected a real change in the underlying amount of disease, related to increased risk factors such as delayed childbirth and the wider use of hormone replacement therapy. But most researchers who tried to explain the phenomenon acknowledged that mammography itself played a big role.[23] (Similarly the recent *decreased* use of mammography may explain the recent *decline* in new diagnoses after 2000, as may the decreased use of hormone replacement therapy.)

There is further evidence for overdiagnosis, but you can't see it in this figure: many of the new diagnoses are ductal carcinoma in situ (DCIS). DCIS is a microscopic breast cancer that, unlike invasive breast cancer, has not spread beyond the duct in the mammary gland. For all practical purposes, there is only one way to be diagnosed with DCIS: have a mammogram. Some doctors believe that DCIS commonly goes on to become invasive cancer; others believe that it does so only infrequently, citing data that suggest less than one-third become invasive.[24] Nevertheless, the clinical reality is that we treat DCIS almost as aggressively as we treat invasive breast cancer.

Only one of the ten randomized trials of mammography provided any information about the value of finding microscopic breast cancers like DCIS. It was the second Canadian study, a study that enrolled women ages fifty to fifty-nine. The control group members each received an annual clinical breast exam, a really thorough clinical exam that was carefully standardized, lengthy (five to fifteen minutes per patient), and generally done by specially trained nurses. The intervention group members each received the same thorough clinical exam each year plus a mammogram. Thus what was really being tested here was the additional value of mammography over that of a thorough clinical exam; in other words, the additional value of detecting abnormalities that cannot be felt. There was no difference in breast cancer mortality between the two groups. To me, this Canadian study conveys an important lesson: there is no obvious value to finding breast cancers that are so small they cannot be felt, such as most DCIS.

But it's important to recognize that overdiagnosis is not simply confined to the diagnosis of DCIS; overdiagnosis of invasive breast cancers occurs as well. A few years ago, I was approached by two Norwegian researchers who had developed a very elegant research design to investigate this issue.[25] They compared two groups of women, both residing in the same Norwegian counties and both fifty to sixty-four years old, over two consecutive six-year periods. One group of 109,784 women was followed from 1992 to 1997, and close to the end of the period nearly all were screened once, as the national screening program began in 1996. This group was the control group. The second group of 119,472 women was followed from 1996 to 2001. All were offered three biannual mammograms as part of the national program, and nearly all accepted. This group was the screened group.

The expectation was that the control and screened groups would have roughly the same number of invasive breast cancers, whether they were detected at the end or found along the way. Figure 6.3 shows what happened instead: the women who had regular screenings had 22 percent more invasive cancers: 1,909 per 100,000 in screened women versus 1,564 per 100,000 in women who did not have regular screening. Although this wasn't a randomized trial, the women were remarkably similar in every way except one: the control-group members got screened once, near the end of the six years; the screened-group members were screened three times over six years. The Norwegian researchers concluded, and I agreed, that this suggested that mammography during the intervening years found some invasive breast cancers that would have disappeared by the final mammogram. In other words, some invasive breast cancers appeared to regress.

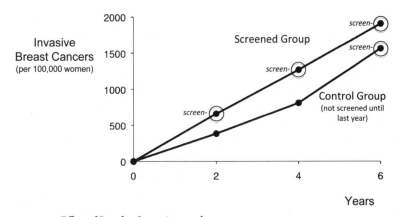

FIGURE 6.3  *Effect of Regular Screening on the Amount of Invasive Breast Cancers Detected*

Overdiagnosis, be it of DCIS or invasive cancer, is a real harm of mammography. Overdiagnosed women are treated for breast cancer. Overdiagnosis is a big part of the reason that women who receive mammography undergo more surgery, not less, than women who don't receive mammography. But look back at figure 6.2; there's more to it than overdiagnosis. The number of breast cancer deaths is going down—there's been about a 25 percent decline since 1990. That's good news. Based on randomized trials, we know that much of this reflects better treatment for breast cancer—particularly tamoxifen and similar anti-estrogen drugs, which have been shown to reduce the risk of death in breast cancer patients by 30 percent. But some of it probably also reflects early detection, specifically mammography. Breast cancer screening involves a trade-off: mammography reduces breast cancer deaths *and* leads to overdiagnosis.

Because overdiagnosis cannot be directly confirmed, its frequency is very hard to measure precisely. Furthermore, the amount of overdiagnosis undoubtedly varies with both the particular radiologist's threshold to label films as abnormal and the particular pathologist's threshold to label an abnormality as cancer. The one randomized trial that does provide long-term follow-up found that, in fact, one in four cancers detected by screening represents overdiagnosis. Remember, most of the remaining three can be treated just as well when they present clinically. But a few will be helped—and helped in a big way: they will avoid a breast cancer death. Our best estimates of the benefit/overdiagnosis trade-off in mammography encompass a wide range: for every one breast cancer death avoided, somewhere between two to ten women are overdiagnosed.[26]

The problem with overdiagnosis is overtreatment. Mammography leads more women to have lumpectomies, mastectomies, radiation, and chemotherapy. It has lead Iona Heath—a physician who is now the president of the Royal College of General Practitioners—to "cheerfully decline" invitations to be screened. She understands the motivation behind early detection. She knows well how terrible a disease breast cancer can be: she has seen women die from it. But she also knows that the ability of mammography to change this fact is rather small. And that there are real harms to the process.

Here's how she summarizes the *Cochrane Reviews'* data:

"The evidence review suggests that for every 2000 women invited to screening for 10 years one death from breast cancer will be avoided but that 10 healthy women will be overdiagnosed with cancer. This overdiagnosis is estimated to result in six extra tumorectomies and four extra mastectomies and in 200 women risking significant psychological harm relating to the anxiety triggered by the further investigation of mammographic abnormalities."

She worries that she has made the decision not to pursue mammography on the basis of information that is not readily available to her patients.

■   ■   ■

IF YOU ARE A NONSMOKING woman, breast cancer is the cancer to be most concerned about. A new breast lump should be investigated with a diagnostic mammogram. Most women with breast cancer will do well (as, thankfully, my wife did). Yet some will die. Given this fact, it is certainly reasonable to consider screening as a way to reduce the risk of breast cancer death. But screening increases another risk—the risk of overdiagnosis.

It has been difficult to have a rational discourse about screening mammography. Many in the cancer community fear that the public can't deal with the reality that screening helps some and hurts others. They worry about sending any messages that might discourage people from getting screened. This may explain why none of the government-run mammography screening programs in seven European countries mentions overdiagnosis in the patient-information pamphlets.[27] But by hiding overdiagnosis, they exacerbate the problem. If the public doesn't know about the problem of overdiagnosis, then all the forces line up to make the problem worse. Radiologists will look harder at images, pathologists will look harder at biopsy specimens—both afraid only of missing cancer, not of overdiagnosis. Medical journals will reflexively conclude that the best test is always the one that sees more, not less. So will the news media.

Of course, these concerns also apply to screening for other cancers. Encouragingly, the prostate cancer experience does seem to be changing the cancer community. There is probably no organization that has pushed more for screening in the past than the American Cancer Society. But their current chief medical officer frequently expresses his concerns about the inevitable problem of overdiagnosis with cancer screening to physicians and the public alike. The Centers for Disease Control now acknowledges overdiagnosis in their decision guide for prostate cancer screening. And the National Cancer Institute's PDQ (Physician Data Query) informs health professionals and patients about the problem of overdiagnosis in screening for a number of cancers. I'm cautiously optimistic that a more balanced discussion about mammography is coming.

Assuming this assessment is correct, I wonder if we might be ready for one more randomized trial. I believe we could reduce the problem of overdiagnosis (as well as reduce false alarms) yet still preserve the death benefit if we were willing to look less hard for breast cancer. The second Canadian trial tells us that screening mammography has no apparent benefit over a carefully standardized physical examination of the breast. But the practical reality is that it is much easier to standardize the practice of the relatively few mammographers in the United States than it is to standardize the practice of the very large number of primary care practitioners who might perform the careful physical examinations (not to mention dealing with the problem of finding the time for them to do so). So I'd like to see a trial comparing current mammography practice with a more conservative one: calling a mammogram suspicious for cancer (and undertaking a biopsy) only if the detected abnormality could plausibly be felt (a size, say, greater than one centimeter).[28]

Cancer screening—the purposeful effort to search for early cancers in those who are well—has led to a lot of overdiagnosis. But sometimes we stumble onto a cancer when we're not even looking for it.

# CHAPTER 7

# We Stumble onto Incidentalomas That Might Be Cancer

SOME FIFTEEN YEARS AGO ONE of my patients, Mr. Baker, called me because he was hoarse. There was no mistaking it—I barely recognized his voice on the phone. I asked him whether he had been sick. He said he felt fine; the only thing bothering him was the hoarseness. I asked him how long he had been hoarse. When he told me it had been about six weeks, I was concerned. The duration of hoarseness and the lack of other symptoms made laryngitis or some other upper respiratory infection unlikely. And although Mr. Baker had quit smoking about three years earlier, he had been a longtime smoker. These two facts made me worry about cancer of the vocal cords or, worse, lung cancer. Lung cancer often involves the lymph nodes near the center of the chest. The nerve to the vocal cords actually loops down from the brain to a point near these lymph nodes before turning upward to the vocal cords. If the nodes enlarge with cancer cells, they can trap the nerve, which, in turn, paralyzes the vocal cords—causing hoarseness.

One of the nice things about a small hospital like the White River Junction VA is that the doctors tend to be able to connect with one another pretty easily. It just happened that the ENT (ear, nose, and throat) doctor had an office down the hall from me. When I got off the phone with Mr. Baker, I walked over to his office, told him about my patient, and asked if he would take a look at his vocal cords for me. He agreed that the procedure should be done and made an appointment to see Mr. Baker. When he examined Mr. Baker's vocal cords a few days later, he found a small tumor that he sent for biopsy. There was no doubt about it—my patient had cancer of the vocal cords. But it was an early cancer. It hadn't spread anywhere in the neck. In fact, most of it had been removed during the biopsy itself. Mr. Baker's hoarseness resolved almost immediately. He was given a short course of radiation and told to come back if his hoarseness returned. That would have been the end of it, except that someone along the way had ordered a chest X-ray.

Now, some doctors might argue that he should have had a chest X-ray anyway, given the possibility of lung cancer. I would counter that once we had found the cancer responsible for Mr. Baker's hoarseness we did not need to go looking for a second cancer. But the horse (my apologies) was out of the barn. Although Mr. Baker's lungs looked fine, the radiologist expressed some concern about a possible widening of the mediastinum, the central region of the chest, between the lungs. Because that widening could represent another cancer, the radiologist suggested a CT scan of the chest.

The CT scan of Mr. Baker's chest was normal. The radiologist concluded that the mediastinum was fine and that the chest X-ray had simply been misleading. But the CT scan had actually gone well below the chest. Because the lungs extend lower in the back than the front, all chest CTs have to include some of the abdomen if they are going to scan the entire lung. The CT had scanned part of Mr. Baker's liver, stomach, and kidneys. And there on the right kidney was a mass just about the size of a golf ball. It was almost certainly cancer. That was a surprise. A patient had called complaining about hoarseness and received a diagnosis of kidney cancer.

I've told this story at a number of physician gatherings over the years, and I always get the same response: laughter. That doesn't mean physicians are uncaring or enjoy hearing about the misfortune of others. Instead, it reflects their familiarity with the absurdity of the situation—we have all been involved in similar diagnostic cascades and stumbled onto abnormalities that clearly have nothing to do with the original problem being investigated. And we are all familiar with the resulting quandary over what to do next.

You may remember that I had once done a small experiment and ordered a sinus film on myself even though I had no symptoms. I was rewarded with a surprise finding of sinusitis. But surprise findings also occur in patients who have symptoms. What makes those findings surprising is that the abnormalities clearly have nothing to do with the symptoms. The typical surprise finding is a small nodule detected on a scan—a patient hears that there is a "spot" on, for instance, the liver, lung, or kidney. Such nodules could plausibly be cancer. But they almost never are. That is why radiologists have dubbed them incidentalomas (*incidental* as in "minor or trivial"; -*omas* meaning "tumors or growths").

Consider these examples:

- A woman gets an MRI of her brain after having an epileptic seizure and is found to have a cyst in her sinus. The cyst has nothing to do with the seizure.
- A man gets an X-ray of his ribs after slipping on the ice and is found to have a spot on his lung. The spot on his lung has nothing to do with his fall.

- A woman gets a CT scan of her lungs because she has trouble breathing and is found to have a nodule in her liver. The nodule has nothing to do with her difficulty breathing.

Surprise findings happen a lot with CT scans and MRIs. Sometimes we do a CT to examine the abdomen but find something in the chest instead, and sometimes we do a CT to look at the chest but find something in the abdomen. While surprise findings are always just that to the patients, physicians see them so often that they aren't that surprising to us.

There is a reason why we get so many surprises: CT scanning reveals minuscule anatomical detail. CT scans consist of a series of cross-sectional X-rays of the human body, with slices scanned as close as every millimeter for that portion of the patient's height under examination (the typical CT will involve between fifty and a hundred and fifty slices, although fewer may be examined by the radiologist). A computer compiles these images and projects them on large video monitors. It allows radiologists to enlarge certain views and change the brightness and contrast to highlight specific organs. They can see abnormalities as small as one to two millimeters—or about as small as the tip of a ballpoint pen.

CT scans have really helped us learn a lot about what's wrong in sick patients. They can show us appendicitis, bleeding in the brain, inflammation in the pancreas, and whether or not cancer has spread to other parts of the body. But, like all diagnostic technologies, CT scans can show too much, detect too many surprise findings, and overwhelm the doctors who interpret them.

### Incidentalomas

The most common incidentaloma is usually found in the lungs. Small lung nodules are detected on chest CT scans in roughly 15 percent of nonsmokers and in up to 50 percent of smokers.[1] The vast majority of these nodules will never become cancer. Neither will the other commonly found incidentalomas, those in the liver, kidney, thyroid, and adrenal gland. But they do pose a problem. One of my closest colleagues, William Black, is a radiologist who has thought a lot about this problem. He estimates that of every ten thousand CT exams, at least a thousand will have one of these incidentalomas.[2] Most of these incidentalomas will never progress to cancer, but one or two will. What should we do? Even if five incidentalomas turned out to be clinically significant, that still leaves 995 overdiagnosed patients. We don't know which patients are in which category. And we really don't know if we can help the five who have cancer. We may or may not have stumbled onto their lethal cancers in time to make a difference.

So should radiologists tell everybody about his or her incidentaloma? Make everybody come back for a follow-up scan? This is what some professional organizations recommend.[3] But it will undoubtedly make many worry needlessly and lead a number of patients to receive unnecessary invasive diagnostic procedures or surgery. And we don't know whether finding an incidentaloma actually helps anyone.

A college and medical-school classmate, a surgeon who must decide whether incidentalomas should be biopsied, recently wrote to me about how he frequently struggles with incidentalomas.

> Twice a month, or so, I see a patient who has had a CT scan done to evaluate some symptom that would have been simply watched before the advent of cross-sectional imaging, and that usually would have amounted to nothing. Typically she is a younger woman: she is healthy, but has had an incidentally detected lesion in her liver. They come to my office, often with additional studies already done. You have seen the radiologist's report—"indeterminate lesion in the liver, cannot exclude metastasis or primary malignancy, suggest MRI." And, of course, the MRI adds absolutely nothing—aside from adding $500–1,000 in cost.
>
> Then they come to me and I have to reassure them that the finding is not cancerous. But what about hepatic cell adenoma—it is not a cancer, but it can become cancer. So, of course, we order follow-up studies. No one wants to defend failing to follow up a possibly malignant lesion in a young woman. So maybe we get a liver biopsy—again, usually equivocal: probably not cancer, but could be—with the risk of bleeding and even death due to bleeding. Or we get 4 or 5 more CTs with the increasing risk of radiation from all the studies both for the women and the eggs in her ovary. Never mind the emotional distress that they all go through.

It's a struggle that more and more doctors have to deal with. We feel trapped by incidental findings. We feel obligated to evaluate them even as we worry that doing so is really not in the patients' best interests. We know they cause a lot of unnecessary worry; we know they add a lot of cost to the system. We also know they lead to more invasive procedures—procedures that pose a real chance of harm, including death. No matter how rare those events are, they do exist. In fact, the chance of dying from the liver biopsy needed to evaluate the incidentaloma (about one to two per thousand[4]) is on the same order of magnitude as the estimated chance that the incidentaloma is a fatal cancer.

### How we know that most incidentalomas are not cancer

I was recently asked by a reporter how doctors know that the vast majority of incidentalomas represent overdiagnosis. It's a good question. At the most basic level, we know that there are far more radiological abnormalities, the reservoir of incidentalomas, than there are people dying from the respective cancers. So much so that we can infer that the chance of an abnormality (like a nodule) becoming a lethal cancer is extraordinarily low. In fact, we can begin to quantify the upper bound of this risk, the highest it could possibly be, using actuarial reasoning that dates from the seventeenth century.[5] Assuming the number of people who die from a particular disease is constant, the probability that a person detected with the abnormality will eventually die from it is inversely related to how often these abnormalities are found. Let's say 10 percent of the population dies from cancer X. Let's also say that 10 percent of the population has incidentalomas suggestive of cancer X. Under these conditions, it's entirely plausible that everyone with that incidentaloma could die from it:

$$\frac{10\% \text{ die from Cancer X}}{\substack{10\% \text{ found to have incidentaloma} \\ \text{suggestive of Cancer X}}} = \frac{10\%}{10\%} = 100\% \text{ could die from incidentaloma}$$

Now imagine we find more incidentalomas. The same 10 percent of the population still dies from cancer X. But now let's say that 50 percent of the population has incidentalomas suggestive of cancer X. All of a sudden it's no longer plausible that everyone with that incidentaloma could die from it. In fact, at most 20 percent of those found to have the incidentaloma could die from it:

$$\frac{10\% \text{ die from Cancer X}}{\substack{50\% \text{ found to have incidentaloma} \\ \text{suggestive of Cancer X}}} = \frac{10\%}{50\%} = 20\% \text{ could die from incidentaloma}$$

Using this reasoning, table 7.1 provides estimates of the highest possible ten-year risk of cancer death posed by various incidentalomas for a typical fifty-year-old.[6]

TABLE 7.1  *Chance that an Incidentaloma Represents a Lethal Cancer for a Typical Fifty-Year-Old[7]*

| Organ | Proportion of People with an Incidentaloma on CT scan (a) | Ten-year Risk of Cancer Death (b) | Chance That the Incidentaloma Is a Lethal Cancer [highest possible] (c = b/a) | Chance That the Incidentaloma *Is Not* a Lethal Cancer (d = 1– c) |
|---|---|---|---|---|
| Lung (smokers) | 50% | 1.8% | 3.6% | 96.4% |
| Lung (never-smokers) | 15% | 0.1% | 0.7% | 99.3% |
| Kidney | 23% | 0.05% | 0.2% | 99.8% |
| Liver | 15% | 0.08% | 0.5% | 99.5% |
| Thyroid (by ultrasound) | 67% | 0.005% | <0.01% | >99.99% |

With the exception of lung nodules in smokers, less than 1 percent of these incidentalomas could possibly represent lethal cancers. So more than 99 percent of the time there is nothing to fix.

Of course, these are just estimates. The second column in particular, representing the proportion of people with incidentalomas, will vary from group to group. These data largely come from a study of over a thousand people who chose to undergo whole-body CT.[8] The data will be different in different populations, particularly in populations with varying ages (incidentalomas become increasingly common as we age, as does the risk of death). And because when we look harder, we find more, these data will also vary based on how carefully the scans are read by radiologists.

The third column, representing the ten-year risk of death, is from U.S. mortality data and—with the exception of separating lung cancer for smokers and never-smokers—reflects the typical American.[9] Some will raise the question of whether an incidentaloma might lead to death in a period longer than ten years. But even if you used a twenty-year time frame (and again with the exception of lung nodules in smokers), it would still be less than 2 percent of these incidentalomas that could possibly metastasize into lethal cancers.

You might reasonably wonder why the data in table 7.1 are the highest possible estimates of the chance an incidentaloma will progress to a lethal cancer in the next ten years. The calculation assumes that *all* lethal cancers develop from incidentalomas that are visible a decade earlier. This is clearly not the case. Other abnormalities can develop over time and eventually result in cancer deaths, further lowering the chance that a specific incidentaloma represents a lethal cancer.[10]

So the numbers above are estimates, but they do give you some sense of the magnitude of the problem that radiologists, and the rest of us, face when finding incidentalomas.

### Follow-up on Mr. Baker

I discussed Mr. Baker's kidney incidentaloma with a number of doctors. Unlike most cancers, kidney cancers are not always biopsied. The reason is that the imaging studies usually tell us what we need to know. And given the images we had for Mr. Baker, the urologists were sure about what to do: take his kidney out. But the radiologist (and I) weren't so sure. This was in the 1990s, and reports about a substantial reservoir of kidney cancer were just beginning to appear in the medical literature. We were also concerned because Mr. Baker's other kidney was fairly small, raising the possibility that he might not do that well with just one kidney.

I presented the dilemma to Mr. Baker. Instead of his having a major operation to remove his kidney, which is associated with an immediate mortality of 2 percent,[11] he and I opted to simply keep an eye on his incidentaloma. This was certainly not standard practice, particularly at that time. Honestly, I think it was easier on Mr. Baker than it was on me and Dr. Woloshin, who took care of him the year I was away on sabbatical. We ordered CT scans of his kidney every six months. On some scans it seemed that the mass had grown a little. I can remember the radiologists measuring it with their calipers and saying it might have been half a centimeter larger. On other scans, it didn't seem to have grown at all.

A few years ago, Mr. Baker died after developing pneumonia. He had an autopsy, which I attended. It was confirmed that he had died from a widespread pneumonia. But I was really interested in his kidney. The five-centimeter (about two inches) mass we had seen on CT was now visible to the naked eye. Viewing a slice of it under the microscope, the pathologist diagnosed it easily: renal cell carcinoma. The pathologist examined tissue throughout Mr. Baker's body, including his brain. Beyond that one in the kidney, no other cancer was found. Mr. Baker had had a diagnosis of kidney cancer for about a decade. He was never treated for kidney cancer, never developed symptoms of kidney cancer, and did not die from kidney cancer. He was overdiagnosed.

I'm glad he never got treatment. It's a big operation, and it could have shortened his life. But I wish he had never gotten that chest X-ray, which led us to get the CT scan, which led us to stumble onto his incidentaloma, which resulted in many years of CT scans every six months and, perhaps more significant, a decade of needless anxiety.

### Kidney cancer—the big picture

It turns out that Mr. Baker's story (or some version of it) has become increasingly common in the United States—common enough to be apparent in national data. Figure 7.1 shows the SEER data for kidney cancer.

It's a picture that should look familiar by now. But there is something different here. This picture is not the product of kidney cancer screening. Instead, it's the product of detailed imaging of other areas, typically CT scans of the thorax, abdomen, or pelvis, that nonetheless detect kidney cancer. In other words, it's the epidemic of incidentalomas.

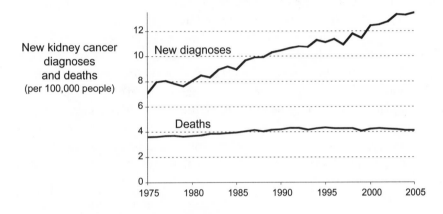

FIGURE 7.1 *New Diagnoses and Deaths from Kidney Cancer in the United States, 1975–2005*

Kidney cancer overdiagnosis is becoming more broadly recognized. A recent investigation in 2009 considered how fast fifty-three kidney tumors progressed. The investigators found that tumors grew at very different rates.[12] Seven (14 percent) actually got smaller—they regressed. Twenty-one (40 percent) grew so slowly that it would take more than six years for them to double in size. That means that, for example, a one-centimeter (0.4-inch) tumor would take more than twelve years to grow to be four centimeters (1.6 inches). Important to note is that these slow-growing tumors were more common in the elderly. Thus a substantial proportion of kidney tumors represent overdiagnosis: either because the tumor doesn't grow at all or because its growth rate is too slow for it to cause symptoms before the patient dies of other causes. Information like this has recently led urologists to recommend that small kidney cancers not be treated immediately but instead followed with serial CT scans to determine if they're progressing fast enough to warrant treatment.[13]

This is clearly a step in the right direction, but I'm not sure following incidentalomas is always the right answer. I think we need to ask a bigger question: should radiologists even call them abnormalities in the first place? The minute they do so, they start a cascade: more testing, more worry, more cost, and—worst—more harm. All most likely for nothing. Although this may feel a little different than choosing the number to define diabetes or hypertension, it is the same basic question: what constitutes abnormal? Medical experts set the bar for what's considered high in blood pressure, cholesterol, and blood sugar; radiologists should decide what's important in abnormalities rather than just reporting any and all of them. Since we are stumbling onto incidentalomas all the time, it's certainly worth thinking about this question.

My view is that we should think of incidentalomas as screen-detected findings. Although we intentionally decide to screen, and we stumble upon incidentalomas by chance, there is no other difference. The patient has no symptoms of cancer. So what we know about screening ought to inform how radiologists react to incidentalomas. To understand what I mean, imagine finding an incidentaloma and asking yourself, *What is the right thing to do for the patient?* (In this exercise, physicians should pretend this is a fantasy world with no lawyers.) Let me show you how I would answer this question under three distinct conditions:

1. *We know screening reduces cancer mortality:* That's easy—I'd call it an abnormality and act on it. We know breast cancer screening reduces breast cancer mortality (at least, among older women), so if an abnormality that looks like cancer in the breast is detected, I'd tell the patient, share the trade-offs with her, and allow her to make an informed choice. Here, there is real benefit to be had. Unfortunately, this is not the typical case.

2. *We don't know the value of screening:* This is hard, and it depends where one thinks the burden of proof belongs. One could argue for calling it an abnormality, telling the patient about it, and engaging the patient in shared decision making (some might say this is the way doctors avoid hard choices), but then some of the harm has already been introduced: the patient has been scared about a possible cancer.[14] Because I think the burden of proof should be on demonstrating the benefit of diagnosis,

radiologists should seriously consider ignoring incidentalomas in this category, effectively dismissing them as too unlikely to be important to be noted in a report.

3. *We know screening does not reduce mortality:* I think that's easy too—ignore it. Don't call it an abnormality; call it normal. Protect the patient from overdiagnosis and overtreatment. Don't mention the finding in the radiology report and don't tell the primary care physician so she won't feel obliged to tell the patient. Again, like *borderline* high blood sugar, cholesterol, or blood pressure, an incidentaloma could be determined by the radiologist as simply too small to be worth noting.

By now, I hope you understand my rationale for this last answer. And I hope it sounds perfectly reasonable. But you should know that it would have radical implications for our current practice in dealing with the most commonly detected incidentaloma: a nodule seen on a chest X-ray.

The diagnosis of a lung nodule is made in hundreds of thousands of Americans each year.[15] It triggers a cascade of follow-up X-rays and scans. More important, it leads patients to worry that they have lung cancer. I have a patient who has been undergoing semiannual scans for years following the detection of a small nodule seen on a chest X-ray that was taken when he had pneumonia. He is constantly worried about what he calls that "spot on my lung." I have not been able dissuade him (or his lung doctors) from this continuing search, an effort intended to determine whether the nodule is growing that also has the unintended effect of making it much more likely that a second incidentaloma will be detected. The effort seems particularly ill-advised since the patient has severe emphysema, a lung disease that precludes his having surgery to remove any cancer that might be found. At least no one wants to take the next step—a biopsy of the lesion—also because of his emphysema. But many patients with nodules do go on to have biopsies.

Unfortunately, the lung is among the most difficult organs to biopsy. A needle is inserted through the chest wall or a fiber-optic scope is placed down the windpipe. Either approach risks puncturing the lung, which can have disastrous consequences, particularly in those with severe emphysema. But we know that lung cancer screening with chest X-rays does more harm than good[16]—that's why no one recommends it and why we don't do it. So why do we do so many follow-up investigations of lung incidentalomas in an effort to cure lung cancer? If we know that chest X-ray screening in general does not reduce mortality, why would pursuing the incidental finding of a pulmonary nodule be more effective? Wouldn't labeling the nodule as normal be the best course of action?

Of course, I'm guilty of oversimplification here. First, there are real-world legal concerns: doctors aren't punished for overdiagnosis, but they are punished for failing to diagnose. So it's hard for doctors to ignore incidentalomas. Second, it's hard to know what is truly a surprise finding. It's not always clear that a symptom has no plausible relationship to a finding. Some findings are ambiguous. If an incidental finding is plausibly related to symptoms, it makes the chance of benefit from further intervention higher (and the chance of overdiagnosis smaller). And, finally, more fine-tuning is possible. We might ignore smaller, less worrisome incidentalomas and those found in patients who have a higher chance of dying from some other disease (like elderly patients or my patient with severe emphysema). For larger, more worrisome incidentalomas in patients with longer life expectancies, we might act, albeit cautiously (for example, by monitoring and looking for evidence of growth before committing to more drastic action).

More and more doctors recognize that following incidentalomas over time is generally a more prudent course than immediate surgery. In fact, protocols are being developed to do exactly this for incidentalomas that are suggestive of lung and kidney cancer.[17] I believe that if we could lower the intensity with which we react to incidentalomas, we'd do better by patients.

■  ■  ■

MOST OVERDIAGNOSIS IS THE RESULT of a purposeful decision. Some organization decides to change the rules about what constitutes an abnormal value, another recommends screening, or an individual doctor chooses to image a part of body to see if he can find an abnormality that might be responsible for a symptom. But no one plans to find an incidentaloma. It is a simply a side effect of doing more scanning at such high resolutions. And while many doctors will argue for the value of lowering thresholds to diagnose conditions or are strong proponents of screening, I don't know of any who believes that finding incidentalomas has been a great advance. Instead, most doctors view them as a nuisance. Many understand that they have become a real problem.

Nevertheless, some doctors may also recall one or two cases in which both they and their patients were convinced that the finding of an incidentaloma had saved a life. These dramatic anecdotes make change more challenging. More important, these stories fail to consider the alternative possibilities: the patient may yet die from his cancer; the cancer may have been every bit as treatable if it had presented clinically; or the cancer had never needed treatment in the first place—the problem of overdiagnosis. The truth is it is very hard to ignore something once it has been found—even if ignoring it is the right thing to do. Doing so will require a huge social and medicolegal shift. It's a lot easier not to do the test in the first place. It is certainly possible not to do a screening test. But there is no way to avoid all diagnostic tests, and no one would want us to (although we could certainly be more judicious in their use). And as long as we are doing diagnostic scans, we will have to deal with the problem of incidentalomas.

Patients could help by being a little less enthusiastic about scanning in general. In particular, they should avoid whole-body scans, which can open a Pandora's box of incidentalomas. They could also be a little more hesitant about other scans and, when given the choice, choose the most anatomically focused exam to avoid stumbling onto things outside of the area of interest. A colonoscopy, for instance, uses a scope to look closely inside the colon for cancer. It examines the colon and nothing else. Recently, there has been growing enthusiasm for virtual colonoscopy, not because it is better than regular colonoscopy but because it is a less invasive exam. A virtual colonoscopy uses a CT scanner to take high-resolution images of the colon, but it also gets images of the liver, the kidney, and even the base of the lungs. And roughly half of virtual colonoscopy exams will reveal abnormalities outside of the colon.

The vast majority of these incidentalomas are not cancer. A few may be. But if we pursue all of them, many will suffer needless anxiety, testing, and intervention. It's just another dimension to the problem of overdiagnosis.

# CHAPTER 8

# We Look Harder for Everything Else

*How Screening Gives You (and Your Baby)*
*Another Set of Problems*

OUR ENTHUSIASM FOR SCREENING EXTENDS well beyond cancer. We screen for abnormalities in your heart and your blood vessels; we screen for metabolic abnormalities (such as diabetes and hypothyroidism); we screen for osteoporosis in your skeleton; and we even screen for abnormalities in your baby in utero. And the tests we use to screen go well beyond images of anatomic organs. They range from sophisticated biochemical measurements that are performed in specialized laboratories to electronic monitoring of basic physiologic functions. But the underlying paradigm of all this screening is the same: We are looking hard to find something wrong because of the belief that early diagnosis—and subsequent intervention—improves health. This paradigm has been applied broadly, so broadly, in fact, that it would be impossible for me to review the screening undertaken for all conditions other than cancer; that would be a book in itself. Instead, I will provide a sample of what modern medicine has to offer.

### Looking hard at the heart's function

In 1985, after working for the U.S. Public Health Service, I continued my medical training as a resident in internal medicine at the University of Utah Medical Center. The university hospital was a technologically intensive setting that was recognized nationally for its expertise in heart disease. Immediately prior to my arrival, the medical center had pioneered the Jarvik artificial heart (an ill-fated device for which there was initially a great deal of enthusiasm and publicity; it was removed from the market in 1990). It was also one of the country's premier centers for heart transplantation. But the technology at the University of Utah Hospital that stands out most in my mind wasn't used to treat heart problems; it was used to find them.

For more than fifty years, doctors have monitored the heart's rhythm using electrocardiograms (or EKGs) in the hospital. EKGs trace the electrical impulses that stimulate the heart to beat so that it can pump blood. Over the decades the electronics of EKGs have been miniaturized, allowing us to monitor patients' hearts while they go about their daily activities. Technology is now so advanced that this information is continuously recorded, allowing us to analyze it later on computers and to quickly summarize the patterns of thousands of heartbeats.

During my residency, the University of Utah participated in a nationwide study called the CAST study (Cardiac Arrhythmia Suppression Trial) that monitored just over seventeen hundred patients who had recently had heart attacks. Following a heart attack, some patients have major disturbances in their heart rhythms. Their hearts may beat much too fast, much too slow, or vacillate between the two extremes. These patients don't feel well. Their blood pressure can drop precipitously and lead to a number of symptoms: they may feel weak or light-headed; they may be unable to stand; they may become unconscious; and some may even die. Patients who had any of these symptoms were excluded from the study. The CAST study focused on patients who felt well after their heart attacks. The investigators were screening for abnormalities in the heart rhythm that were silent, those the patients would never have known about without heart monitoring. Researchers were concerned that asymptomatic abnormal rhythms, primarily extra heartbeats, might portend more lethal rhythm disturbances. The investigators wanted to see if early diagnosis and treatment of asymptomatic abnormalities could prevent sudden death in the year following the heart attack.

Although the investigators envisioned that monitoring would eventually be done at patients' homes, the study was initiated in the hospital in order to standardize the process. A heart attack patient who was doing well and was ready to be discharged was first sent to a special unit and attached to a small heart monitor. The job of responding to the monitor's findings fell to the medical residents like me.

It drove us nuts. The patients were well, but their monitors were always going off. It seemed as though every one of them had an abnormality. And we were treating them. We were constantly adjusting medications to try to find the right drug and the right dose to make the rhythm normal. Occasionally, it seemed as though what we were doing was working. But more often, our efforts didn't seem to make any difference. And sometimes what we did seemed to make matters worse. Many of us thought the whole effort was crazy.

It was. CAST was a randomized trial. The medication given to about half the patients was a placebo. In other words, we were functionally ignoring the monitor findings in around 850 patients. This turned out to be the right thing to do; they fared better than the treatment group. After a two-year period, the trial was stopped because it had become evident that the drugs were not preventing lethal rhythm disturbances but actually causing them: the death rate in treated patients was two and a half times higher than in those given a placebo. The investigators tried once more, this time focusing on the most severely abnormal heart rhythms and using another drug (the CAST II trial), but again more patients died in the treated group.[1]

This was one of the first studies that made me wonder whether looking hard for things to be wrong might be a mistake. If you have a disturbance in your heart rhythm that is severe enough to cause symptoms, you should have it diagnosed and treated. But looking hard for silent electrical abnormalities in the heart and treating them is a different matter entirely.

The heart isn't the only muscle stimulated by electrical impulses. The nervous system uses electrical impulses to spur the contractions of every muscle in the body. We can therefore monitor the activity in any muscle we choose, including the uterus. The uterine walls contract during labor, a normal process unless it happens too early. Premature birth is a major cause of infant illness, injury, and death. With five hundred thousand babies born prematurely in the United States each year, some doctors hoped that early diagnosis of premature uterine contractions followed by treatment to stop them could prevent some premature births.

In the early 1990s, Kaiser Permanente of Northern Californian initiated a randomized trial examining the value of monitoring the uterus in about twenty-four hundred pregnant women at high risk for giving birth prematurely.[2] The two most common risk factors were carrying twins, which are often born early, and having a prior history of premature labor. Women in the intervention group were given home uterine monitors and were told to use them for one hour every morning and evening. They were instructed to immediately transmit the information by telephone to an obstetrical center. The center personnel evaluated the information, and when faced with worrisome results that suggested premature contractions, they told the women to seek medical care. To ensure that the women followed this protocol, the intervention group also received daily calls from nurses.

The women in the control group were simply contacted weekly. They were not given uterine monitors; there was no effort made to detect early signs of labor. The study, which took place over four years, found that monitoring naturally led to more medical care: monitored women were almost twice as likely to have unscheduled visits with their obstetricians than unmonitored women (2.3 visits on average, as opposed to 1.2 visits) and were 50 percent more likely to be treated with drugs to suppress uterine activity than women in the control group (19 percent of the treatment group women were treated, as opposed to 12 percent of the control group). But monitoring had no effect on the rate of premature birth: 14 percent of women in both groups delivered early. So all the extra diagnosis was overdiagnosis; all the extra treatment was overtreatment. Home uterine monitoring is no longer considered a part of standard obstetrical care.

### Looking hard at your baby's heart function

Now we can also monitor the electrical impulses of a baby's heart in utero during labor. The procedure typically involves placing a belt that contains an ultrasound device around the expectant mother's abdomen. Electronic fetal monitoring has been performed for nearly fifty years in an effort to ensure that the fetus is getting enough oxygen during labor. If it's not, the baby's heart rate often slows down considerably. When an obstetrician sees a slower heart rate on the monitor, she may decide to deliver the baby immediately with an emergency cesarean section. A C-section is the surgery to remove the baby through the mother's abdomen. It's a big operation. A slow fetal heart rate on the monitor does not lead to a planned operation—that's an elective C-section—it leads to an emergency C-section in a woman who had been trying to deliver vaginally. And as is true for most operations, C-sections have higher surgical risks when done emergently. The situation is less well controlled, the personnel are less ready, and the operation has a higher chance of complications.

The Cochrane Collaboration, an independent international organization dedicated to consolidating research about the effects of health care, has been summarizing studies of electronic fetal monitoring for years. After reviewing experimental studies involving more than thirty-seven thousand women, they haven't found much evidence that monitoring leads to benefit. Fetal monitoring doesn't appear to make babies any healthier at birth, as measured by their Apgar scores, the standard evaluation of a newborn's appearance, pulse, grimace, activity, and respiration. Nor does it reduce the number of newborns who develop cerebral palsy, have to go to the intensive care unit, or die.[3] The only benefit the researchers found was a lower risk of seizures in infants who had had fetal monitoring, down from about two seizures to one seizure in every thousand births.

But as you might have guessed, monitoring does lead to far more emergency C-sections. In the Cochrane summary, monitoring increased C-section rates by 66 percent. And C-sections are a lot more common than seizures, particularly in the United States. Applying these data to the United States (where four of the twelve studies were done), it means that monitoring is responsible for escalating the frequency of C-sections from about 200 in every 1,000 births to 330 in every 1,000 births.[4]

Figure 8.1 compares the benefits and harms of electronic fetal monitoring.

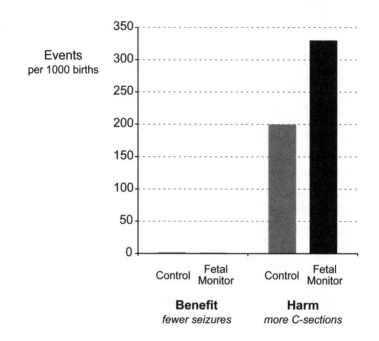

FIGURE 8.1 *Effect of Intrauterine Electronic Fetal Monitoring*

No, that's not a misprint. The figure looks blank on the left because seizures are so rare relative to C-sections (but trust me, the difference between the two seizures per thousand births without fetal monitoring and the one per thousand with it is there). To be fair, it is not entirely clear how one can compare seizures with C-sections; they are like apples and oranges. But it is clear that there is a huge trade-off involved in implementing electronic fetal monitoring: it takes 130 C-sections to avoid one seizure. The other 129 cases represent overdiagnosis: these babies were diagnosed with abnormally slow heart rates that didn't require emergency C-sections.

In 1996, the U.S. Preventive Services Task Force, the independent panel of experts that reviews screening tests, recommended *against* routine fetal monitoring.[5] But according to their current Web site, fetal monitoring has become such an ingrained fixture of medical care that, frankly, the task force seems to have simply given up on trying to dissuade doctors from using it:

Despite the lack of evidence on its positive impact on health outcomes and the 1996 USPSTF recommendation against its routine use, intrapartum electronic fetal monitoring in pregnancy has become common practice in the U.S. Based on currently available evidence, the USPSTF believes there would be limited potential impact on clinical practice in updating the 1996 recommendation. The USPSTF will not update its 1996 recommendation.

Fetal monitoring is indeed an ingrained fixture of medical care—the last time the federal government examined the topic, in 1999, electronic fetal monitoring was used in 83 percent of all U.S. births.[6]

### Terrifying pregnant women

Pregnancy is not a disease, but increasingly doctors are treating it like one. No one has precise data on routine obstetrical practice in the United States. While we have excellent national data on health care for elderly Americans because of the Medicare program, there is no equivalent organization that tracks what happens to pregnant women. What information we do have suggests that common practice no longer includes home uterine monitoring, but it does regularly include electronic fetal monitoring during labor and another screening test, obstetrical ultrasound.[7]

Having an ultrasound, also known as a sonogram, has become a routine part of pregnancy. At the same time that the federal government last surveyed the use of fetal monitoring, they also documented that 64 percent of women have at least one ultrasound during the pregnancy. Instead of using X-rays, the imaging uses sound waves at a frequency so high that they cannot be heard by the human ear (that's why there is an *ultra-* before the *sound*). Ultrasound produces a remarkable image of the fetus, which is undoubtedly the major reason why expectant parents like the test. But it is still a screening test. It is looking for something wrong with the baby, even though there is no reason to believe there is anything wrong.

When she was pregnant, Dr. Schwartz came across an article entitled "Obstetrical Sonography: The Best Way to Terrify a Pregnant Woman." When she showed it to me, I suspected it came from some back-to-nature periodical or an alternative-medicine publication. But it wasn't; it was from the *Journal of Ultrasound in Medicine*, the official journal of the American Institute of Ultrasound in Medicine. And the author wasn't some outside critic of sonography but a consummate insider, Dr. Roy Filly. Dr. Filly is a professor of radiology and of obstetrics and gynecology at one of the country's top medical centers, the University of California at San Francisco (UCSF) School of Medicine. For years he has directed their section of diagnostic ultrasound. He performed some of the first obstetrical ultrasounds almost forty years ago. And this is what he wrote in the article Dr. Schwartz and I found so surprising at the time:

> The opportunity to say, "Everything looks fine" to an expectant mother was one of the perks of my job. I can see the wave of relief wash across her face. It's always a touching moment followed by "thank you, Doctor."
>
> Today, I no longer feel that way. There are a growing number of patients where I dread having to speak to her. I have reviewed the sonographer's scans and they disclose a finding that will send the mother into a tailspin of confusion and worry. . . . Tomorrow when I return to work the odds are I will have to speak to a mother-to-be about an "abnormality" that I see on her sonogram and I won't know what to tell her.[8]

Over the last few decades researchers have published volumes of scientific papers on the anatomic abnormalities associated with trisomy syndromes, a feared class of genetic defects. The name comes from the fact that there are three copies of the chromosome in question instead of the usual two; Down syndrome is the most familiar trisomy syndrome, but there are a number of others. The problem is that the anatomic abnormalities associated with the genetic disorders—such as "bright spots" in the heart or intestine— aren't all that abnormal. While they are found in fetuses with trisomy, they are also common in normal fetuses. Dr. Filly estimates that around 10 percent of normal fetuses will have at least one of these "abnormalities."

The trisomy syndromes are pretty rare—all together they occur in only three out of every thousand live births.[9] But the anatomic abnormalities occur in 10 percent of normal fetuses, or a hundred of every thousand live births, so if we do an ultrasound on every pregnant woman, there's going to be quite a lot of overdiagnosis. For every hundred fetuses found to have abnormalities, three at most will actually have trisomy.[10] The other ninety-seven are overdiagnosed—diagnosed as having an abnormality when, in fact, the "abnormality" is of no consequence. But once women are told about the abnormal findings, there are substantial consequences. There's a lot more testing, more amniocenteses, and more miscarriages (published estimates of amniocentesis-induced miscarriages range from 0.06 percent to 1 percent[11]). And perhaps more important, pregnant women are terrified during what should be one of the greatest experiences in life.

For Dr. Filly, this is an important problem that affects his patients in a most immediate way:

> The physicians in the trenches read these scientific papers and then identify these "abnormalities" during a routine sonogram. What are they to tell the patient? This woman hasn't already been counseled. She is having a sonogram for "reassurance" (forget that now). Her husband, children and parents are with her. There is a party atmosphere. The videotape is rolling. Soon the giggling and finger pointing at the screen will cease. The questions will change abruptly from "is that the heartbeat?" or "is that the penis there?" to "are you saying that my child is going to be mentally retarded?"
>
> Without doubt you have now added cost to the management of that pregnancy. The patient may choose to undergo amniocentesis. She may be referred to a prenatal diagnostic center for a detailed fetal sonogram and genetic counseling. The innumerable hours of counseling by primary care givers and general sonologists to explain the "meaning" of this finding are not counted in these additional costs. Nor are the heartaches of the parents-to-be counted in this cost analysis. If they forego the amniocentesis (clearly the correct choice, in my opinion) then they must live with residual doubt for the remainder of the pregnancy. Does my fetus have Down syndrome? Maybe I should have had the amniocentesis. The enjoyment of the anticipation of the birth of their son or daughter is now replaced with anxiety.
>
> Well you say, look at all the good these findings have accomplished. Some bad must go along with all that good. Possibly I am the exception (I doubt it), but I don't see "all the good." I am a simple-minded physician. . . . From my vantage point the identification of these "abnormalities" in low risk women has crossed the line of "more harm than good."

You should know that Dr. Filly is not the exception. A major review of fifty-six studies of these abnormalities concluded that they were not reliable enough indicators of trisomy for clinical practice. The authors of the review stated that using these ultrasound-detected abnormalities to screen for trisomy would actually lead to more miscarriages than diagnoses of trisomy syndromes.[12]

In pregnancy, overdiagnosis is a diagnosis given to a pregnant mother who would otherwise deliver normally or given to a fetus destined to be born a healthy infant. The fetus (or mother) in fact has the abnormality being sought, but it would otherwise have no consequence. In our health-care system, we are eager to make diagnoses and often do so under the guise of preventive measures for those who are perfectly healthy. Given the advances in technology, it should come as no surprise that we often make diagnoses in utero in fetuses, some of whom do in fact have genetic disorders, but many of whom are healthy. Our enthusiasm for early diagnosis extends to pregnancy. Home monitoring led more women to be told that they were going into preterm labor than ever did. Fetal monitoring suggests that more fetuses are suffering from a lack of oxygen than in fact are. And in both cases our zeal for diagnosis leads to additional unneeded interventions, either more drugs to stop labor or more emergency C-sections.

Fetal ultrasound abnormalities are an even more peculiar case. These findings generally do not trigger treatment interventions, but instead more diagnostic interventions and more unnecessary anxiety. Some of my colleagues might consider them to be not overdiagnoses but rather false alarms, or what we call false-positive tests. Most of the time, however, false alarms are recognized to be false fairly quickly, typically by a subsequent test. Fetal abnormalities detected by ultrasound aren't usually resolved by further testing. Because more definitive tests simply don't exist, aren't that definitive, or are avoided because they increase the risk of miscarriage, fetal ultrasound abnormalities aren't discovered to be spurious until a healthy child is delivered. While I acknowledge that there is room for legitimate disagreement about exactly how to label this problem, to me it seems to be yet another example of overdiagnosis.

And I think that is what most women who have experienced the problem would say. Ultrasounds can detect a lot of other abnormalities—abnormalities that have no association with the trisomy syndromes. The diagnosis of any abnormalities can terrify parents about their baby's future. *New York Times* science reporter Natalie Angier wrote about the fallout from a routine ultrasound examination twenty weeks into her pregnancy, an experience that is not uncommon:[13]

> I had enjoyed the sonogram. Expectant parents do. It is a bonding opportunity. It is baby's first video. I had already had amniocentesis several weeks earlier, to check for chromosomal abnormalities associated with so-called elderly gravidas like my 38-year-old self.
>
> I knew that my baby had 23 neatly matching pairs of chromosomes, that her spinal tube had closed and that she did not have a gruesome defect like anencephaly—no brain—that would propel me to have an abortion despite having struggled for years to get pregnant.

In sum, I knew my baby was healthy and magnificent, and had gone into the ultrasound expecting added proof of her splendor.

The obstetrician began discussing the scan results. Her tone was hesitant, clipped, distinctly not the voice of reassurance. A siren of panic began wailing in my skull. She said this was fine, that was fine, blah, blah, blah. Come on! I thought angrily. Get to the point! What's wrong with my baby?

Finally, the doctor came to the problem. The left foot. She said the results were difficult to interpret. The foot was in a funny position in the uterus, crammed down deep in the pelvis, so it could be simply a matter of its position at the moment. But the sonographer had not been able to see the profile of the foot, no matter what angle she came at it from, and that is what happens when you have a clubfoot. My husband and I looked at each other in dumb, grim shock. Clubfoot? Neither of us was sure what a clubfoot was, what it looked like or how bad a defect it was. The term was so thuddingly ugly and Dickensian that we could not help imagining the condition must be ugly and severe.

The obstetrician told us we had a couple of choices. We could go to a university facility for a more in-depth sonogram, or we could just do nothing and go on with the pregnancy. A clubfoot would not affect the course of the pregnancy, she said, and any effort to correct it would have to wait until after the baby was born.

Oh, sure, do nothing and forget all about it—that is a realistic option, I thought bitterly. Thus we started down a rutted path trudged by so many tens of thousands of people each year, that of medical testing and retesting, the contemporary version of consulting the Oracle of Delphi or a platter of entrails. It is a path that is getting bumpier and more perilous by the month, as ever more high-tech assays are added to the list of prognostic options. . . .

Leaving the obstetrician's office, my husband and I headed for a medical library to do research on clubfoot. The pictures in textbooks were devastating. Some of the feet were extremely deformed, bent in and up at the ankle to form the letter J. Toes and heels were bunched and twisted. The feet were often stunted, and the calves of the clubfoot leg were comparatively underdeveloped. . . .

That night, my husband and I did not sleep at all. We wept and wept. Privately, we each pleaded with the universe to make the follow-up sonogram come out normal. We offered up our own body parts in exchange: eyes, arms, feet.

The universe was deaf. The next day, a doctor at a nearby university hospital concurred with the preliminary diagnosis of clubfoot, subtle though the evidence was. "Good catch!" he said admiringly of the previous sonographer's work.

In the car ride home, I howled so hard I thought the sky would crack; but the sky stayed whole and calm and blue.

A week later, we met with a genetics counselor at a different university to discuss the odds that the clubfoot might not be an isolated defect, but part of a larger genetic syndrome. We had yet another sonogram, performed by doctors with extensive expertise in ultrasound diagnosis. Happily, they were able to rule out larger genetic anomalies, but of the clubfoot they were certain. "There is a varus deformity of the left foot," they said bluntly.

I became obsessed with clubfoot, medically and culturally. I learned that for several months to a year our daughter would have to wear a thigh-high cast designed to twist her foot gradually into a normal, usable position. I learned that the cast would have to be changed every week, that casting alone might not work, and she might require one or more operations. As for the asymmetry of her calves, that would be untreatable and permanent. . . .

I also spoke to mothers of children with clubfeet and was inspired by their stories. They assured me the casts in no way slowed their children down or interfered with motor milestones like crawling. They said that with their feet fixed, the children could walk and run with the best of the nonclubbed masses. Finally, toward the end of my pregnancy, I began to relax.

In late August, I gave birth to a healthy daughter with a lusty set of lungs, a full head of black hair—and no clubfoot at all.

Routine ultrasounds may bring joy to and reassure, sometimes falsely, millions of parents. But they also scare numerous others. And it's not clear they do much else. The Cochrane Collaboration found no substantive benefit to routine obstetrical ultrasound. In fact, it appears to lead to more C-sections; although the mechanism is not clear, the additional testing may simply raise the anxiety level of both physicians and mothers. The psychological impact of all this testing on mothers has been poorly studied.[14]

In 1996, the U.S. Preventive Services Task Force recommended *against* routine obstetrical ultrasound.[15] Their current position is that, just as with fetal monitoring, there would be little use in updating the recommendation.

Ultrasonography in pregnancy has become routine practice is U.S. medical care. Here's what they now write:

> Despite the lack of evidence on its positive impact on health outcomes and the 1996 USPSTF recommendation against its routine use, ultrasonography in pregnancy has become common practice in the U.S. Based on currently available evidence, the USPSTF believes there would be limited potential impact on clinical practice in updating the 1996 recommendation. The USPSTF will not update its 1996 recommendation.

Sound familiar? It's exactly what they wrote about fetal monitoring.

### Vascular screening

In the last few years, there has been a lot of enthusiasm for so-called vascular screening. Doctors are increasingly looking for abnormalities in the major blood vessels, blockages in the legs (known as peripheral artery disease), blockages in the neck (carotid artery stenosis), and aneurysms in the abdominal aorta. These abnormalities are all related. They all reflect the common underlying disease of atherosclerosis, and they all share a common risk factor: smoking. The definitive treatment for each is surgery.

These screenings are widely promoted by commercial ventures, such as Lifeline, Prevention Health Screenings, and Legs for Life. They are for-profit companies who advertise their ability to make early diagnoses and save lives. Often, these vascular screenings are packaged with a screening test for a completely unrelated disease, osteoporosis. Increasingly, the vascular tests are also being promoted by academic medical centers. The University of Pennsylvania, the University of Maryland, Georgetown, Columbia, and even my own center, Dartmouth-Hitchcock, all provide vascular screening.

These screenings detect a number of abnormalities, turning the people who undergo them into new patients who need additional follow-up exams, enhancing diagnostic-testing revenues. Some will have definitive therapies, enhancing procedural revenues. But while vascular screenings may serve financial interests, they almost certainly do not serve the interests of public health. In fact, with the exception of abdominal aortic aneurysm screening in men who are or have been smokers, these screening tests are at odds with the recommendations from the U.S. Preventive Services Task Force.

The task force recommends *against* screening for peripheral artery disease, carotid artery stenosis, and abdominal aortic aneurysms in women. It has no recommendation for abdominal aortic aneurysm screening in men who have never smoked, and recommends one screening test only for those aged sixty-five to seventy-five who have. The task force recognizes that many of the new patients identified by screening are overdiagnosed. They are made to worry needlessly. Some will receive treatment that cannot help them but that nonetheless entails substantial risk.

Even the best of these screening tests, the one for abdominal aortic aneurysm, is a delicate balance between benefits and harms, as shown in table 8.1.[16] It reflects several studies involving more than a hundred and twenty thousand men age sixty-five and older, about half of whom were screened and half of whom were not, and shows what happened to both groups during the course of five years.[17]

TABLE 8.1  *A Decision Aid for Men Considering Undergoing Screening for Abdominal Aortic Aneurysm*

| AAA Screening: Benefits and Harms | | |
|---|---|---|
| | **After Five Years:** | |
| | **Among 1,000 men *not* screened for AAA** | **Among 1,000 men screened for AAA** |
| **Did AAA Screening help?** | | |
| Number of men who died from abdominal aortic aneurysm | 3.4 | 1.9 |
| Difference in deaths from all causes combined | 14 | 14 |
| **Did AAA Screening have downsides?** | | |
| Number that required a major operation to repair aneurysm | 5 | 11 |
| Number that required an indefinite cycle of follow-up testing triggered by screening | 0 | 55 |

Screening reduced the five-year probability of dying from a ruptured aneurysm by almost half. But because that probability was low to begin with, only 1.5 men per 1,000 screened experienced this benefit (3.4 – 1.9). And screening had no effect at all on the overall risk of death, which was the same in both groups.

For every man who avoided an aneurysm death because of screening, three were treated for naught—in other words, underwent surgery unnecessarily. As always, surgery poses harm, such as heart attack, blood clots, and potential damage to the circulation to the legs, kidneys, and intestines. Of course, some portion of those three may benefit at some point beyond five years (the life expectancy of a sixty-five-year-old is about seventeen years), so there's no way to be certain whether they were overdiagnosed or not. At the same time, more than 5 percent of men who were screened were told that the aorta was abnormal but not sufficiently so to require immediate surgery. Instead, they were informed that they needed surveillance, or follow-up testing, possibly for years. Some of these men will eventually be told they need surgery. So there is likely to be more overdiagnosis to come.

How would you react to being told you have an aneurysm but one that's not yet serious enough to require surgery? What is it like to undergo surveillance every six months, say, over many years? Men contemplating screening should know about the anxiety experienced by this group. One of my vascular surgery colleagues, Brian Nolan, interviewed thirty-four men undergoing surveillance at our center and found that many do worry: 7 percent of men reported difficulty falling asleep, 25 percent felt overwhelmed, and 48 percent reported unwanted thoughts about the aneurysm. But how some men really feel about knowing they have an AAA (and undergoing surveillance) is best communicated using their own words: "Daily I feel as though little to nothing is being done for my condition"; "My family is much more concerned with it rupturing than I am. They treat me like I'm an invalid and won't let me lift anything"; "I don't let my grandchildren sit on my lap"; "I feel like I am carrying a bomb that could explode at any time."

There's no right answer. AAA screening will help a few, but will lead many more to worry needlessly.

■    ■    ■

COMMON MEDICAL PRACTICE IN THE United States now includes screening for all sorts of disorders. It is a natural extension of the zeal for early diagnosis. More and more people are told they—or their babies—have abnormalities. Of course, some are helped. But sometimes we know that the number who benefit from screening is extremely small, and sometimes it is so small we can't even measure it in large studies involving tens of thousands of patients. More often we are not sure if screening has any benefit at all. But we persist on focusing intently on early diagnosis and quite often fail to consider overdiagnosis.

# CHAPTER 9

# We Confuse DNA with Disease

*How Genetic Testing Will Give You Almost Anything*

I REALLY LIKE THE SCIENCE of genetics. In high school, I enjoyed calculating the probabilities of various genotypes using the simple genetics Gregor Mendel discovered cultivating pea plants. In college, I was fascinated to learn how the selective pressures exerted by one very common infectious disease (malaria) actually favored the persistence of particular genetic diseases in human populations (sickle cell disease, glucose-6-phosphate dehydrogenase deficiency). And in medical school, I was intrigued by the mechanics of DNA: how the double helix is replicated, how it gets transcribed into RNA to make proteins, how it gets recombined so we can pass on some of our mothers and some of our fathers to our children, and how it can get usurped by other life forms (viruses) so that our cells work for them.[1] Genetics is a wonderful mix of mathematics, evolutionary biology, and biochemistry. It's good stuff.

But I am much less enamored of the idea of testing healthy people's genes. Some think that genetic testing will provide a road map to optimal health. Genetic testing is already useful in helping us tailor therapy to individual cancers and is likely to become more useful in predicting how well patients will respond to various drugs. And gene therapy—treatment for a specific disease that involves altering DNA itself—could, in certain settings, prove to be a genuine medical cure. But genetic testing could just as easily be a road map to widespread ill health.

Already, numerous commercial enterprises exist that will take your DNA (and your money) and tell you about your future. One such company, 23andMe, promises to "unlock the secrets of your own DNA," while Navigenics wants you to be tested and "do everything you can to stay healthy." And deCODEme hopes that genetic testing will "prompt people to do the right thing." This commercialization of genetic testing appears to be selling health, but from my standpoint at least, it's selling overdiagnosis. Genetic testing of healthy people is the most extreme manifestation of early diagnosis. Here the diagnosis being sought is not a disease but rather the underlying genetic predisposition for a disease. In short, genetic testing is looking for genetic risk factors. Because everybody is at risk for *something*, it's a strategy that will make literally all of us sick.

We already have genetic tests to screen for the predispositions to a lot of diseases—more than I could possibly cover here. And because we are in the midst of an explosion of genetic research, we will undoubtedly have even more tests by the time you are reading this. But the fundamental questions about genetic testing will not change. They are the same ones that should be asked about any early diagnosis effort: How many people will needlessly be told that they are somehow abnormal? What will we do to them?

### *The vision: a baseline genome scan*

Imagine that one day every young adult will have a baseline genome scan, a series of genetic tests that reveal the risk of developing major problems like heart disease, psychiatric disorders, diabetes, and cancer. Now imagine that you are a healthy twenty-year-old woman who is having her first genome scan. You spit into a special cup—that's right, your genes are in your saliva— and mail it to one of several genetic-testing companies. A couple of weeks later you receive an e-mail announcing that your personal risk profile is complete. You open the report.

**Baseline Genome Scan for:** Ms. Smith

| Disease | Your Genome Scan | Your Lifetime Risk of Developing Disease | How Your Risk Compares with the Average Person's |
|---|---|---|---|
| Ovarian cancer | OvXX *present* | 8.5% | 4 times greater |
| Lung cancer | LNx5 *absent* | 0.5% (if nonsmoker) | About half average |
| Breast cancer | Bc59y *present* | 17% | About 1.5 times greater* |
| Heart disease | CHDmd21 *present* | 40% | 1.25 times greater |
| Macular degeneration | CHDmd21 *present* RetinX76 *absent* | *net effect unknown* | Less than average Higher than average |

* There is considerable debate about the accuracy of this estimate in the medical literature.

The risk profile shown above suggests that you have an 8.5 percent chance of developing ovarian cancer sometime in your life. That's four times greater than average. Fortunately, you don't have the gene that is strongly associated with an increased risk of lung cancer in both smokers and nonsmokers, so we know that your risk of developing that disease is well below average. But you do have a gene that some researchers believe increases your risk of breast cancer by almost 50 percent, although the report notes that there has been considerable debate about this estimate in the medical literature recently.

The profile shows that your risk of heart disease is 1.25 times average, and you are reminded that you need to take that seriously since heart disease is by far the most common cause of death in the United States. (This finding doesn't really surprise you, because your mother had a heart attack a couple of years ago, and you know that family history is often a good indicator of your risk for disease.) One of the genes that raises your risk of heart disease also happens to lower your risk of macular degeneration, a disease that leads to a progressive loss of vision. But then again, you also have a different gene that raises the risk of macular degeneration. You are told that researchers are actively working to better quantify these relationships, but for the time being this is the most accurate data they can provide.

Some road map. It doesn't show you how to get to optimal health. It doesn't even tell you what you can do to improve your chances of remaining healthy. Nor does it warn you about the road hazards that may lie ahead: more testing, more overdiagnosis, and more intervention. While this might sound like science fiction, it's not. Most of these tests are available now, and those that aren't could be soon, given the explosion of current research. The vision of a baseline genome scan was first articulated over a decade ago by Francis Collins, the head of the Human Genome Project. In his annual report to Congress in 1998, Collins wrote, "A baseline genome scan could give patients and health care providers helpful information about an individual's disease risk profile and point to which prevention strategies—when available—should be put into place."[2] While it's tempting to think that more information about your predisposition to develop certain diseases can only help you, there can be real hazards to having this information.

I can remember making a similar statement when discussing the Human Genome Project with the father of one of my childhood friends. I really respected this man: he was an attorney in charge of a large municipal airport and he always enjoyed an energetic political discussion. He said that my concern about having more information smacked of my being "anti-science." That hurt. I felt like he was accusing me of being a biblical literalist, arguing that Copernicus was wrong and the earth was indeed the center of the universe, or arguing against evolution at the Scopes monkey trial. But it did help me think about an important distinction: the difference between knowing more about the science of human genetics and knowing more about your own particular genome. The two are separate issues. I'm all for pursuing the science, but I worry greatly about the unintended side effects of personal genetic testing—side effects that stem from our thinking we understand more than we do. To better grasp the hazards of knowing more about your personal risks, you need to have some idea of how our medical culture reacts to this information.

### More testing, more intervention

A diagnosis that suggests you are at high risk for particular diseases has serious consequences. It gets everybody (you, your family, your doctors, and maybe even your insurance company) worrying about the bad things that are just waiting to happen. This anxiety typically translates into more testing, which will in many cases detect more expected "disease" as well as some surprise findings, which triggers more intervention: medication certainly, and possibly surgery.

A woman with the breast cancer gene may start getting mammograms earlier than she would have otherwise (such as at age thirty-five instead of age fifty) and more frequently. In addition to increasing the potential for overdiagnosis, earlier and more frequent mammography exposes women who are already predisposed to breast cancer to more radiation. Similarly, a man with the prostate cancer gene may start getting PSA tests earlier (such as at age forty instead of age fifty) and more frequently. In either case, because genetic information suggests that the patient is at high risk, doctors will have a much lower threshold for performing biopsies. And as you now know, this increased testing invariably leads to more diagnosis, more overdiagnosis, and more intervention for breast or prostate cancer. Furthermore, if the testing involves images that extend beyond the organ of interest (as happens with CT scans), unexpected findings may be detected. They lead to more intervention as well.

Simply finding out that you are at high risk may lead directly to intervention of another kind: interventions to prevent the disease. The woman who is told she is at elevated risk for breast cancer may take tamoxifen to lower her risk or may even undergo a mastectomy as a preventive measure. The man who is told he is at elevated risk for prostate cancer may take finasteride or undergo a prostatectomy as a preventive measure. The central problem with genetic information is uncertainty—uncertainty about who will in fact get the disease and what should be done about it now. Much of this uncertainty will always be with us, no matter how well we understand human biology.

### *Genetics is not destiny*

The information contained in genes is often described as the blueprint for the human body, although some scientists feel that the more appropriate analogy is to a recipe, which turns out a little different each time. There is a gene with a set of instructions responsible for eye color, another with instructions for how to make insulin, and another with instructions that may or may not enable you to roll your tongue. And you have about twenty-five thousand others. Genes are composed of only four building blocks, whose names are abbreviated with the letters A, C, G, and T. The code is formed by stringing these building blocks together; the average gene has three thousand building blocks (the range is from 252 to 2.4 million). The vast majority—over 99 percent—of this genetic information is identical in all of us. This makes sense, since we all have so much in common: we each have two eyes and one heart (with the same four chambers), we each walk erect, and so on. But the small amount of genetic information that does differ from person to person really matters. It's a big part of what makes people different from one another.

In the simplest case, genetics would be completely deterministic. Genes alone would be solely responsible for individual characteristics. But genetic variation is not the whole story. Even identical twins, who have exactly the same DNA, or genotype, are not exactly the same. Environmental factors, particularly in early life, also matter. Things like nutrition and harmful exposures to toxins or radiation affect human characteristics, even before birth, as does physical and intellectual activity in childhood. There is a broad scientific consensus that virtually all variation is the result of the interaction between genes and environmental factors. And then there is luck, or the random play of chance. The same genotypes in the same environment may still yield quite different people.

This leads to a key distinction that is relevant to genetic testing: the distinction between genotype and phenotype. The complete set of genetic instructions contained in your DNA is your genotype. The human that others can observe—your physical, biochemical, and behavioral characteristics—is your phenotype. You don't experience your genotype; you experience your phenotype. And it is the combination of your genotype, your environment, and luck that determines your phenotype.

Genetic testing attempts to predict your phenotype based solely on your genotype. While there's really no reason to have a genetic test to predict an aspect of your phenotype you already know about—you wouldn't, for example, do a genetic test to see if you had blue eyes—some genetic-testing companies are in fact promoting tests just like this. They claim they can test your genes to see whether you have trouble tolerating milk products, or whether you have problems with ear wax, or even whether you like Brussels sprouts.

There really is a gene associated with liking Brussels sprouts. Let's say you don't like Brussels sprouts. Maybe you have the gene, maybe you don't. While your genotype is a major factor in developing your phenotype, it's not the only one. Maybe your parents taught you not to like Brussels sprouts. Or maybe your only experience with the vegetable was in hot lunches in the high school cafeteria. Maybe you have never had well-prepared Brussels sprouts— freshly harvested, lightly steamed, and then sautéed with garlic, mustard, and walnuts (somehow I never did during my first three decades of life . . . sorry, Mom). But if you don't like Brussels sprouts, do you really care whether this preference is mediated by your genes or your environment? And if you do like Brussels sprouts, would you stop eating them if you found out that you were missing the liking-Brussels-sprouts gene? Geneticists are the first to point out that phenotype trumps genotype.[3]

### *Abnormal gene does not equal disease*

The only compelling reason to test the genotypes in healthy individuals is to predict their future phenotypes, specifically, whether or not they will develop particular diseases (or pass them on to their children). But what is true for individual characteristics is also true for diseases. While some diseases are determined solely by the presence or absence of specific genes, most reflect the interaction among genetics, environment, and pure chance. The public (not to mention doctors) can fall into the trap of equating a genetic abnormality with a disease. Certainly, some genotypes predict which individuals develop certain phenotypes almost perfectly, but others are weak predictors at best. The measure of how well genotype predicts phenotype is called penetrance, or the frequency with which a particular gene produces its effect in a group of individuals.

Few genetic abnormalities have a penetrance approaching 100 percent. One classic example is cystic fibrosis, an illness that appears in childhood and affects the secretions of the lungs, liver, pancreas, and intestines. Most people with the disease do not live past forty. Cystic fibrosis is an autosomal recessive genetic disease. If you inherit the abnormal gene from just one parent and get the normal gene from the other, you are a carrier but won't develop the disease. But if you are unfortunate enough to inherit the abnormal gene from each of your parents, then you are almost certain to develop the disease.[4]

Another example of a definitive genetic abnormality is Huntington's disease, a degenerative neurologic disorder that appears in midlife and leads to jerky, random, and uncontrollable movements, as well as impaired cognitive function. There is no known therapy. Huntington's disease is an autosomal-dominant genetic disease: you need only inherit the abnormal gene from one parent to develop the disease. In Mendelian genetics, Huntington's disease is another classic: an autosomal dominant disease with virtually 100 percent penetrance.

The penetrance of most genetic diseases, however, is substantially less than 100 percent. Even the powerful breast cancer–associated genes BRCA1 and BRCA2 predict a risk, not a certainty, of developing breast cancer. Estimates of their penetrance range from 30 percent to 70 percent. [5] To be clear, that's the chance of developing the disease by age seventy, not dying from it. Because these estimates tend to come from women who have both the genes and strong family histories of breast cancer, the genes themselves may have less penetrance in women without family histories. And not having BRCA1 and BRCA2 doesn't mean you won't get breast cancer. In fact, your risk is still about average—approximately a 10 percent chance of developing the disease by age seventy—because the vast majority of breast cancers, more than 95 percent, have nothing to do with the BRCA genes.[6] They are instead sporadic, reflecting the interaction of other risk factors and the role of chance.[7]

Many disease genes have even lower penetrance. There is a spectrum, going from definitive genes to highly penetrant genes to weakly penetrant genes. And the more we learn about the genome, the more we recognize that definitive and highly penetrant genes are relatively rare, and that most genetic information is only weakly related to the development of disease.

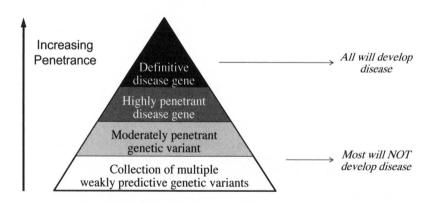

FIGURE 9.1 *The Spectrum of Disease-Gene Penetrance*

This spectrum of penetrance is beginning to affect the language geneticists use to describe genes. Some feel that the term *gene mutation* implies certainty and should therefore be reserved for highly penetrant genes. For genes with lower penetrance, geneticists prefer the terms *gene variant* and *genetic aberration*.[8] At the bottom of the spectrum are gene variants that are so poorly penetrant that we need to combine the results of testing multiple variants (at different points on the genome) to make any reliable prediction about phenotype.

While we are learning more about the genome every day, most of the new information is about weakly penetrant genetic variants. The reason is simple: definitive disease genes have been obvious for decades. We didn't have to read human DNA to understand the genetics of cystic fibrosis and Huntington's disease. The genetics for these diseases were deduced in the 1930s and 1870s, respectively. [9] Definitive disease genes are the low-hanging fruit of genetics, obvious simply by studying family trees. If your father, your father's father, two of three brothers, and half your cousins all have a rare disease, it's fairly obvious that there is a genetic basis for the disease. Most of what we are discovering now is much less obvious; the genetics for the diseases are not evident in family trees. Instead, their effect is apparent only in carefully designed studies involving hundreds or even thousands of individuals.

Overdiagnosis and penetrance are inversely related. The less penetrant a gene is, the more overdiagnosis will occur, because most people with low-penetrance genes will not in fact go on to develop the disease.

### Case study: A genetic disease affecting iron metabolism

Hereditary hemochromatosis is a genetic disease that leads to the excessive absorption of dietary iron. The excess iron accumulates throughout the body, in the heart, liver, pancreas, adrenal glands, and musculoskeletal system. It is the kind of disease we hated to learn about in medical school: it has too many manifestations. Patients might present with heart failure, cirrhosis of the liver, diabetes, adrenal insufficiency, arthritis, or just a general feeling of malaise. And there are a lot of other diseases that can produce similar problems. As students, we felt that everything about hemochromatosis was complex and vague. Because it was associated with so many symptoms, it could almost always turn up on a list of possible diagnoses for a patient. Hemochromatosis is the kind of disease that makes young doctors want to avoid the complexities of internal medicine and specialize in cardiology or go into surgery, where the problems are more straightforward.

But at least the treatment was pretty straightforward. If you want to get rid of iron in the body, all you need to do is bleed the patient. That's right: the standard treatment for hemochromatosis was and is to this day blood-letting. Bloodletting, or phlebotomy, is a therapy with a sorry history in medicine. For more than a thousand years, doctors withdrew considerable amounts of blood in the belief that doing so cured a variety of maladies. In fact, losing blood is bad for virtually all sick patients[10]—unless, that is, they have hemochromatosis. The reason bloodletting helps patients with hemo-chromatosis is simple: red blood cells contain a lot of iron. Removing them with therapeutic phlebotomy forces the body to make more red blood cells. And making more red blood cells requires removing iron from existing iron stores, thereby lowering the amount of iron in the body.[11] So there is not a lot of debate about how to treat hemochromatosis. But there is con-siderable debate about how to diagnose hemochromatosis.

Hemochromatosis was first recognized to be a hereditary disease in the 1930s, some sixty years before the specific genetic defect was identified.[12] There are actually a number of genetic mutations that can cause hemochro-matosis, but the most common, C282Y, was discovered in 1996. The genetics of C282Y are pretty interesting. It's a defect in a gene that instructs the pro-duction of a protein that regulates iron storage. Because hemochromatosis is an autosomal recessive disorder, to develop the disease you have to inherit the genetic defect from each of your parents—just like cystic fibrosis. The disease variant and normal gene differ by just one building block—there is an A where there should be a G—out of almost ten thousand building blocks in the gene. This defect is believed to have originated from a chance muta-tion in a single Viking ancestor in northwestern Europe some two thousand years ago. It doesn't affect reproductive capacity and may even confer some advantage by providing resistance to iron deficiency, particularly in men-struating women. That may be the reason the mutation has persisted across multiple generations.

Genetic testing for hemochromatosis has certainly made the lives of doc-tors more complicated. Now we have to consider when to seek the diagnosis, as illustrated in figure 9.2. Should we do so when your genotype is knowable, which conceivably could be before you are born—in fact, the moment you are conceived? When you develop the biochemical abnormality of iron over-load (the asymptomatic phenotype), or later when you develop symptoms of the disease (that is, heart failure, cirrhosis of the liver, diabetes, adrenal insuf-ficiency, arthritis, or a general feeling of malaise)?

The existence of three possible diagnostic strategies has produced a fair amount of debate in the medical community about which is the right ap-

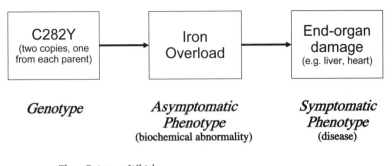

FIGURE 9.2   *Three Points at Which Hemochromatosis Could Be Diagnosed*

proach. The typical diagnosis involves a patient who presents with fatigue, malaise, and painful joints and is subsequently found to have high iron stores. Some have advocated earlier diagnoses: screening for the asymptomatic phenotype of iron overload. It's a simple blood test measuring the proteins that absorb or store iron. Others have advocated genetic screening: testing people for C282Y, as well as other genetic variants, routinely. The debate is consequential enough that the U.S. Preventive Services Task Force decided to weigh in with their recommendation. In their systematic review of the medical literature, they found that, unlike cystic fibrosis, the C282Y gene does not have 100 percent penetrance. In fact, they recognized that the concept of penetrance itself was far more complicated. It was not clear whether *penetrance* should refer to the probability that the gene will lead to the symptomatic phenotype (disease) or to the probability that it will lead to the asymptomatic phenotype of iron overload.

They considered both probabilities and determined that penetrance was incomplete both from genotype to asymptomatic phenotype and even more so from genotype to symptomatic phenotype. Less than half of those inheriting C282Y from both parents develop the biochemical abnormality of iron overload, and less than half of those with iron overload go on to develop the clinical disease.[13] Figure 9.3 presents a more accurate picture of the disorder.

In short, among four people found to have inherited C282Y from both parents, roughly three will not go on to develop the disease hemochromatosis. So if we screen for this genotype, 75 percent of people with the genetic abnormality will be overdiagnosed.

Now one might reasonably argue that we could accept that three patients were overdiagnosed if it was clear that the one who was destined to develop the disease would benefit from early diagnosis. Of course, it would be equally reasonable to argue that patients ought to be able to decide whether or not

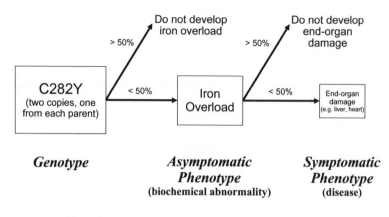

FIGURE 9.3 *Hemochromatosis Penetrance*

to be screened. They could make their own decisions about how to weigh the potential benefit of early diagnosis of genuine disease against the potential harm of overdiagnosis, such as loss of insurance or unnecessary bloodletting. But for the one patient who will eventually develop hemochromatosis to benefit from genetic testing, early treatment must clearly be better than treatment administered when the diagnosis would be made based on symptoms. The task force could find no evidence at all that earlier treatment would help the few who were destined to develop the disease. And because the disease is relatively rare, to find that one person, roughly a thousand people would have to be genetically tested—leading not only to three individuals being overdiagnosed, but also to others experiencing false alarms of being diagnosed incorrectly as having the gene. The task force strongly recommended against screening, concluding that the potential harms for genetic screening outweighed the potential benefits. So for now, at least, bloodletting is not going to reemerge as a common therapy.

### Developing genetic tests for common cancers

Hemochromatosis is a pretty rare disease. It's not the reason so many people are enthusiastic about genetic testing. The real interest lies in determining the risk of common chronic diseases such as diabetes, heart disease, and cancer. Cancer seems to have garnered the most interest by far. We already have a pretty good idea of who is at high risk for diabetes and heart disease. There is no need to do a genetic test to learn about the common, powerful risk factors for diabetes: obesity, sedentary lifestyle, and family history. Nor is there genetic testing needed for heart disease, which has the powerful risk factors of smoking, high cholesterol levels, high blood pressure, diabetes, and family history. But cancer is different. Smoking is the only common, powerful risk factor, and only for some cancers. And nonsmokers get a lot of cancer.

Most cancers seem to be sporadic, almost random. While there are single cancer genes that cause cancer, like the BRCA1 and BRCA2 genes for breast and ovarian cancer and the familial adenomatous polyposis gene for colon cancer, these are responsible for relatively few cancers overall. Most breast, ovarian, and colon cancers have no readily identifiable genetic basis. The same is true for other cancers. Nevertheless, there is a lot of enthusiasm (and a lot of funding) for trying to better delineate the potential genetic contribution to common cancers. And why not? This sort of research seems so appealing. If we could determine who is likely to get cancer, we could start treating them differently and potentially save more lives.

There are two problems with this approach. This first is that it's not clear how to treat them differently. Do we just look harder for cancer to appear—with all the attendant problems associated with this strategy? Or do we actually do something—start a drug or perform a surgery? The truth is: it's very hard to know. And to do research on the best approach requires thousands of patients followed over decades.

The second problem, of course, is overdiagnosis. We may tell way too many people they are at high risk for cancer. They may not only worry needlessly, but also receive tests and treatments that can do nothing but hurt them.

### *Looking harder for cancer risk*

Researchers have taken a new tack in their search for the genetic contribution to common cancers. They know that there will most often be no obvious single gene that causes cancer (such genes would be plainly obvious in family trees), so they have been considering the role of multiple genes in cancer's etiology. Often they are not sure what these genes are, where they are, or even whether they exist. But despite all of this uncertainty, they have got quite a clever approach. They are looking for snips. *Snips* is the phonetic pronunciation for the abbreviation *SNPs*—single nucleotide polymorphisms. A snip is a genetic variant in just one building block of your entire DNA. So if most people have a particular section of DNA that reads AATGGGC and yours reads AATTGGC, you have a snip.

Everyone's genome is full of snips. A few occur in the middle of a gene and affect its function (like C282Y for hemochromatosis). But most snips are in junk DNA, or DNA that has no known function. Some of the junk DNA may represent evolutionary artifacts that served a purpose at an earlier time but no longer do now; some of it may act as a repository of genetic variation that may be useful in the future; and some of it may have a function we don't yet recognize. It turns out that most of our DNA is junk. So even though we all have lots of snips in our genotypes, it hardly matters because most snips don't affect our phenotypes.[14]

Snips are relatively easy to find. Researchers can quickly compare individual genomes and locate the snips. Snips are like unique signposts on the genome, signposts that may be associated with nearby functional DNA (the part of DNA with the genes). Snip patterns are like barcodes in this sense. Even though most snips don't do anything, it's possible their patterns can identify something about the functional DNA, and therefore about the potential to develop various diseases. To determine if snip patterns predict cancer, researchers compare the patterns of snips in hundreds of patients who have the cancer being studied with those of hundreds who do not. Then they fire up some really big computers to determine a formula representing the best combination of snips to distinguish between the two. In other words, you gather genetic barcodes from a large population and see if you can write a barcode formula that can differentiate those who have cancer from those who don't. It's serious statistical work, work that would never be possible without modern computers.

### Case study: Snips and prostate cancer

The prototypic study of this genre appeared in the *New England Journal of Medicine* in February of 2008.[15] The upshot was that a combination of five snips could help predict a man's risk of developing prostate cancer. The study actually tested men with and without prostate cancer for sixteen snips in total. Although all sixteen had previously been found by other researchers to be associated with prostate cancer, this study showed that three of the snips in fact had no relationship with the disease. This study highlights an important caveat about this approach: we now have the ability to read so many snips that some will appear to be related to diseases simply by chance. Remember, most snips don't code for anything and are not themselves responsible for cancer. Instead, they are statistically associated with cancer, and some statistical associations happen purely by chance. So before believing a purported snip-disease association, you'll want to see it replicated in multiple studies.

The researchers went on to choose the five snips most strongly related to prostate cancer. Nonetheless, individually, each of the five snips in this study was (in the authors' own words) "only moderately associated with prostate cancer"—meaning that whatever genes each reflected were weakly penetrant. So the researchers chose to examine the cumulative effect of having multiple snips. The result was an apparently powerful association: men who carry four or all five of these snips have 4.5 times the risk of developing prostate cancer. The researchers were quite enthusiastic about their work. Their press release boasted "for the first time, this type of study has made it possible to develop a clinically viable gene test." And they decided to form a company to market their test to the public.

But their potential consumers need to have a little healthy skepticism about what *viable* means in this case. It could mean that the test is able to be done. Or it could mean it's worth doing. And of course, we are interested in determining the validity of the latter assertion, even if the researchers aren't.[16]

So suppose you are a man with the bad snip barcode, meaning four or all five snips. You're told your risk of prostate cancer is 4.5 times greater. But 4.5 times greater than what, exactly? It turns out that the comparison group used in this study was men without any of the snips. But snips are common. Most of us have them. It's the rare man who has none of the five snips. In fact, only 10 percent of the men in the study managed to have zero snips. If you want an accurate risk assessment, the relevant comparison should be to the typical man in the population, and the typical man has two snips.

As shown in table 9.1, the comparison group used to calculate the degree of risk matters a lot.

TABLE 9.1  *Changing Comparison Groups and Prostate Cancer Risk*

| Number of snips | Prostate cancer risk compared with men at lowest risk (**0 snips**) | Prostate cancer risk compared with a "typical man" (**2 snips**) |
|:---:|:---:|:---:|
| 0 | Comparison group | 50% lower |
| 1 | 1.5 times higher | 25% lower |
| 2 | 2 times higher | Comparison group |
| 3 | 2.2 times higher | 1.1 times higher |
| 4 or more | 4.5 times higher | 2.3 times higher |

Because the comparison group reported in this study was made up of men with zero snips, anyone with any other number of snips will be found to be at elevated risk. So you are led to believe that a man with two snips has double the risk of developing prostate cancer. But, in fact, a man with two snips is at average risk. And the pertinent risk, the risk we are truly interested in knowing, must be assessed using this typical man for comparison. Only then can other test results increase or decrease risk, and no one will have his risk increased 4.5-fold. Instead, as you can see from the table, the biggest change is either roughly doubling or roughly halving the risk of an average man.

Of course, getting prostate cancer isn't the same as dying from it. With the advent of prostate-specific antigen screening, we are beginning to tap the large reservoir of this disease in the general population, undoubtedly detecting and treating some men unnecessarily. In other words, many of the men who develop prostate cancer don't have the kind of disease that kills them. Genetic testing is not likely to solve this problem. Some of the men with prostate cancer in the snip study had very aggressive cancers; others had very indolent cancers. But the snips could not distinguish between the two. The snips could not predict which healthy patients would develop prostate cancer at a young age or which patients had cancers that had already spread beyond the prostate. They could not predict the Gleason score, the pathologist's measure of how aggressive cells look under the microscope, or the PSA level, the biochemical measure of cancer aggressiveness. They did not even predict who had a family history of prostate cancer (surprisingly, since one would expect this information to be contained in the genome). So while the test seemed to help predict the risk of developing prostate cancer, it didn't predict which patients would get aggressive prostate cancers, the type that might be fatal, and which would get prostate cancers that would never go on to produce symptoms.

The risk information it provides is not especially helpful. Simply telling men that they are at higher risk for developing prostate cancer is a recipe for more overdiagnosis and overtreatment. The snips can't tell us what we most need to know: who is at high risk for prostate cancer death.

Yet it is entirely possible that a subsequent study will identify a set of snips that predict prostate cancer death. Imagine that this was the study that did it. Some men would be told their risk of prostate cancer death had roughly doubled; others would be told their risk was cut in half. But by far the most common test results would be smaller changes in risk: 1.1 times higher; no change; or 25 percent lower. All this information—doubling and halving risk and so on—is relative. Relative risk is used to compare the risk in two different groups of people—its usefulness depends on how many people actually have the disease, how rare or common it is. You might be doubling a big number, or you might be doubling a small number. That number, absolute risk, is the average risk of developing a disease over a specific period. Table 9.2 gives you a brief summary of the two measures and a specific type of absolute risk: lifetime risk.

TABLE 9.2  *Relative, Absolute, and Lifetime Risks*

| Measure | Description | Example |
|---|---|---|
| Relative Risk | The most familiar risk expression; actually, it's a ratio of two absolute risks (one relative to the other) | *Mr. X's risk of prostate cancer death is twice that of the average man.* |
| Absolute Risk | The chance (probability) that something will happen. To be complete, an absolute risk must also include the time frame the probability refers to. | *The typical fifty-year-old American man has a 1 in 1,000 (or 0.1%) chance of dying from prostate cancer in the next ten years.* |
| Lifetime Risk | The absolute risk over a specific time—the remainder of your life | *The typical American man has a 3% chance of dying from prostate cancer during his life.* |

The absolute risk of prostate cancer death over a lifetime—the lifetime risk—is roughly 3 percent, so the typical man has a 3 percent chance of dying from prostate cancer. Assuming we had a genetic test that was able to predict prostate cancer death, here's what it might look like: If you have four or more snips, your lifetime risk is 2.3 times higher than 3 percent, or 6.9 percent. If you have none of the five snips, your lifetime risk is half of 3 percent, or 1.5 percent.

No matter how many snips you have, your chances of dying from something other than prostate cancer will always be over 90 percent.

Now imagine a man in his twenties being told he has four or more snips. What should he do differently? Would a lifetime risk of 6.8 percent be high enough to warrant definitive therapy, a prophylactic prostatectomy? Given the risk of impotence, most young men would probably avoid this option. Should he start hormonal therapy? Probably not. It can cause erectile dysfunction and male breast enlargement. So that leaves him with the option of trying to detect the disease in its early stages: PSA screening. And the truth is there's still uncertainty about whether PSA screening reduces deaths from prostate cancer. Nevertheless, many men (and doctors) believe that it does. But if you are a believer, wouldn't you continue to be tested regardless of whether your risk is 6.8 percent, 1.5 percent, or anywhere in between? And if you are not a believer and are worried about the overdiagnosis and overtreatment initiated by PSA screening, will these small changes in your risk change your mind about screening? The major limitation of genetic tests is that their results will have at best a relatively small effect on the estimated risk of experiencing future health events, and certainly not enough of an effect to change what you would (or should) do anyway.

## *"Now what?"*

The question about what to do with the information provided by genetic testing is a significant one. Consider the hypothetical twenty-year-old woman receiving her first genome scan. Her relative-risk profile showed a fourfold increased risk of ovarian cancer, a decreased risk of lung cancer, and a debatable increase in the risk of breast cancer. She also faced an increased risk of heart disease and had genetic variants that both increased and decreased her risk of macular degeneration. We have a lot of information but no guidance as to what we should do with any it. So now what? Some might argue that the first step would be to deal with the fourfold increased risk of ovarian cancer, perhaps by removing her ovaries. Others might point out that the absolute risk for ovarian cancer is in fact quite small. The lifetime risk for ovarian cancer death for the average woman is about 1 percent, so this woman's lifetime risk is still only 4 percent. Some might argue that heart disease would be a more likely cause of death for her, even though she is only at average risk (the lifetime risk for heart disease death for an average women is over 20 percent). Removing her ovaries and disrupting the production of estrogen would only increase her risk of heart disease. Another doctor might suggest removing her ovaries and starting estrogen replacement.[17] But someone else would surely point out that this procedure will increase her risk of breast cancer. These uncertainties, combined with the absence of the lung cancer aberration, tempt her to start smoking.

What's the right thing to do? She shouldn't start smoking; that, I'm afraid, is the only point all the doctors would agree on. Ironically, genetic testing that demonstrates a person has a lower-than-average risk for a particular disease poses its own problems: the potential for the individual to get a false sense of immunity and neglect the most important health behaviors. What to do about the rest of this information—well, the truth is that we don't know.

Our ability to read the genome is well ahead of our ability to know whether medical intervention based on such a reading makes sense. Genetic risk is, after all, only one factor among many contributing to disease (remember, it's nature, nurture, and luck). Thus, while intervention might help a few of those destined to get the disease, it will undoubtedly lead others to be treated for diseases they will never develop, or that will never produce symptoms.

Learning what, if anything, should be done with genetic information will take a long time. It requires large studies spanning multiple decades and involving tens of thousands of people with each genetic variant, some of whom receive intervention and some of whom don't. For some variants, intervention may prove to be of value. For others, it will hurt more than it will help. Often, the findings will simply be unclear, and researchers will call for more studies. But don't hold your breath for the answers. We may *never* know how to implement the results of genetic testing in medical interventions because the nature of innovative processes in medicine can make it impossible to *ever* know. Medical theories rarely remain constant over a period of multiple decades, the time span necessary to carry out longitudinal studies. Changing definitions of disease and the rapid evolution of treatments create a catch-22 scenario in which ideas and technologies come in and out of clinical practice long before clinical science catches up with definitive answers about what works. The only certainty about genetic screening is that overdiagnosis is a built-in problem.

### Why testing cancer genomes may not solve the problem of overdiagnosis

Thus far I have focused exclusively on testing the human genome of a specific individual in an attempt to predict his or her likelihood of developing specific diseases. But there is now considerable enthusiasm for testing the genome of individual cancers—not the person's genome, but the genome of his or her cancer, since a cancer has its own genome, different than that of the patient it resides in. Remember, it is those mutations that make it a cancer.

Some believe that we can decode all of the genetic information contained within individual cancers and that this will finally allow us to determine which ones are aggressive and kill, and thus warrant therapy, and which ones will never go on to cause problems and are better left alone. This approach would appear to solve the dilemma of overdiagnosis, allowing us to select only those cancers that are life-threatening for treatment, but while the concept is promising, it is hampered by serious obstacles.

It turns out that most types of cancer have more than one pattern of genetic mutations. Far more. To reliably predict the prognosis of a certain set of genetic mutations in any given cancer requires observing multiple cancers with the same pattern. But there are so many patterns that there may be too few cancers with the same pattern to observe. This problem of genetic variability among cancers was well encapsulated in the title of a presentation given at a recent conference at the National Cancer Institute: "50,000 Tumors, 40,000 Aberrations."[18] The unfortunate reality is that the genetic information within cancers may be too variable to predict the future of any one cancer.

Similarly, to reliably predict the prognosis of cancer patients—that is, to know which have noninvasive cancers and are better left alone—we would need to observe numerous patients diagnosed with cancer and not give them any treatment. It's been done, largely in studies of prostate cancer. But it would be very hard to recruit enough people with each type of cancer and with each mutation pattern for that cancer who would be willing to forgo treatment long enough to reliably demonstrate exactly how the cancer will behave.

But suppose we had enough cancers and enough willing patients to predict the future behavior of each mutation pattern. We would still be up against another problem: the genome of a cancer can change. In fact, in many ways, a changing genome is a defining feature of cancer: cells rapidly divide and haphazardly replicate their genomes, with mutations accumulating with time. Because cancer genomes are inherently unstable, a test of your cancer's genome today may not reflect your cancer's genome tomorrow. Thus the predicted course of your cancer may well change. And cancer, like all diseases, is about more than just genes. Remember: the same DNA can produce different phenotypes in different environments. How your cancer behaves reflects not only its genome but also something about the environment in which it lives—the host environment within you. So even if we could read the cancer's genome perfectly and predict how it might change in the future, a completely different set of unknowns still remains.

I want to be clear: testing cancer genomes will be useful in selected settings. It is likely that a small subset of genetic variants in some cancers will have a sufficiently high effect on future risks to be identifiable and useful. My guess is, however, that this genetic information will predominantly affect decisions about how aggressively to treat (for example, if we should add chemotherapy following surgery). To solve the problem of unneeded treatment in overdiagnosed patients, we need a test that addresses a more basic question: Do we need to treat at all?

■   ■   ■

ALTHOUGH MOST OF US HAVE normal phenotypes, virtually all of us harbor genetic abnormalities. Each of us can be shown to be at high risk for some disease. So the new world of personal genetic testing has the potential to make all of us sick and arguably poses the greatest threat of overdiagnosis. It's very likely that scientists have already found all the genes that definitely result in a person getting a specific disease, such as the genes for cystic fibrosis and Huntington's disease. And they have probably found nearly all of the genes that, while not definitive, are very powerful predictors of disease, such as the BRCA genes. Now they are searching primarily for gene variants with far smaller effects, variants that marginally increase or decrease one's likelihood of developing cancer, heart disease, diabetes, age-related macular degeneration, and so on. Just what we are predicting is not always clear. And what to do about what we predict is even less so.

Of course, the impact of all this overdiagnosis directly depends on what we do with the information. If we didn't tell anybody anything, no one would do anything differently and there would be no problem. But that would make the test pointless. Perhaps we could ignore all the little changes in risk and communicate only the few really big ones. Then we could focus our research efforts on learning what interventions truly help the people at highest risk.

While that would be the best scenario, I fear it won't happen. The problem is that it is very hard to ignore information. Once you know there is something wrong with your health, there is a great pressure to do something. And if it's not clear what you should do, you can bet this information will lead to a series of haphazard interventions with unknown benefits and unexpected harms. Not to mention that the information can make a lot of people anxious about their health.

But is informing the well about their risks for disease really the road map to a healthy society? Is it healthy for the young to focus on their likely causes of death years before it occurs? And genetic testing doesn't need to be delayed until age twenty; it could be initiated in children, much like cholesterol screening, or even as part of prenatal testing. There is no reason we couldn't learn about a person's risks of death before he or she was even born.[19] Ironically, the healthiest populations may be those that know nothing about their DNA.

# CHAPTER 10

# Get the Facts

A LOT OF MESSAGES ABOUT health screening are simply variations on the same theme—in one form or another, they all push the idea that the best way to stay healthy is to look hard for things that might be wrong. Sometimes the messages reflect the best of intentions: disease advocacy groups and some doctors advise people to be screened because they believe it is right thing to do. Others times they reflect more self-serving motives: health-care companies, hospitals, and some doctors advise people to be screened because they are in the business of selling the service. But regardless of the underlying motivation, what you really need to know is whether these messages are supported by good hard facts.

I should start by telling you the unfortunate reality: all too often, there won't be any good hard facts to find. There is a reason for this. Most healthy people will not soon (or ever) develop the particular disease we are trying to diagnose early. So getting reliable information about the value of early detection for the few who will get the disease requires studying a lot of healthy people for a long time. And a big, long study is a very expensive study. The numbers are impressive: a typical randomized trial of mammography, for example, enrolled around fifty thousand women, followed them over a decade, and cost tens of millions of dollars. Not surprisingly, there are not a lot of these studies, although there should be. The millions we would pay to study the value of early detection pales in light of the billions we spend putting it into practice without knowing if it helps.

But since there aren't a lot of good hard facts out there, it is important to recognize when you are being led to believe that people know more than they do. Many messages about early detection—advertisements, public service announcements, health Web sites, and even news reports—are plainly misleading. They typically exaggerate the risks you face as a way to scare you into taking action. If the benefit of an early detection is not known, the people who are pushing it tend to assume it is beneficial; if there *is* a known benefit, they tend to exaggerate it, using phrases like X *prevents* Y when X *reduces the risk of Y* would be more accurate. Particularly misleading is the frequent misuse of survival statistics, such as five- and ten-year survival, that are known to be horribly biased in the context of early detection. And messages advocating specific screenings often include powerful personal anecdotes: people whose lives were apparently saved by early diagnosis. What the messages don't do is disclose the alternative possibility: these people were, instead, overdiagnosed.

Messages directed at the public, those that seem to be full of good hard facts, can actually be quite deceptive. They are designed to convince you of the benefit of early detection, not to give you a balanced presentation of benefits and harms.

### The new test that finds everything

Let's start with an ad for a hospital that ran in a local newspaper in New England. A young woman, apparently in her thirties, is pictured gazing contemplatively, her arms crossed somewhat defensively. Perhaps she is worried about the news her doctor has just delivered. The ad boasts simply:

*Our hospital found the breast cancer that "wasn't there."*

Is finding the cancer that wasn't there good news? It must seem that way to the hospital's marketing department. But how many abnormalities detected like this represent overdiagnosis? Finding a breast cancer that "wasn't there" probably means that the cancer could not be seen using a standard test (such as a mammogram) but could be seen with another test (such as a contrast-enhanced MRI). So it must have been hard to find: a small abnormality. And if mammography can find cancers not destined to cause symptoms, imagine what an MRI can find.

This brings us to a more general principle about how to think about cancer screening. It's tempting to assume that the best test is the one that finds the most cancer. But the goal is not to find more cancer. The goal is to save lives. And the only way to know if the screening is saving lives is by doing a randomized trial. It is easy to forget this and assume that if technology can find more cancer, it will save more lives. Marketers exploit this assumption. Don't fall for it.

### The scary story

Now imagine you are flipping through a magazine and stumble onto another ad, this one from a nonprofit foundation. A young woman with long flowing hair and deep blue eye look cheerful in a portrait she might have sketched herself. She has written, "It won't happen to me. I go to the gym every morning. I walk to the office. And I don't let work stress me out." And then the tagline:

*Alecia Fox, 21, the day before she was diagnosed with thyroid cancer.*

That's scary. A young woman, the picture of health, is completely unsuspecting the day before she is diagnosed with thyroid cancer. Not only does it scare you about getting thyroid cancer—after all, you might have it and not even know—but it suggests that you are crazy if you are not scared; at the bottom it says "Confidence kills. Thyroid cancer doesn't care how healthy you are. It can happen to anyone, including you." It suggests you "ask your doctor to check your neck."

There is a whole series of these ads. But none of them tells you much about the disease or the benefits and harms of early detection. They instead evoke fear to initiate action and assume you'll think the action is beneficial. So suppose you want to learn more. You go online and find a Web site about the thyroid posted by the American Society of Endocrinologists.[1] There, you learn that "thyroid cancer is one of the fastest growing cancers in America and one of the most curable."

This statement suggests two things: (1) thyroid cancer is a big problem ("one of the fastest growing cancers in America") and (2) we can fix it ("one of the most curable"). The combination of "big problem" and "fixable" seems to make the argument that there is a reason to get screened.

The first part is factually correct: thyroid cancer is one of the fastest-growing cancers in America in terms of the rate of growth in new cases. But it is still relatively uncommon: fewer than two in a thousand people will be diagnosed with it in the next ten years.[2] And no one with a broad view of public health would suggest that thyroid cancer is a big, growing threat to Americans. Over the past thirty years, the death rate from this cancer has not changed. The big, growing threat is not from thyroid cancer but from thyroid cancer overdiagnosis.

The second part of the message—that thyroid cancer is one of the "most curable" diseases—is even more misleading. It is true that patients with thyroid cancer do extremely well relative to other cancer patients. But the word *curable* suggests that this is *because* of medical treatment. But when you consider the possibility of overdiagnosis, you recognize an alternative interpretation—for some, there was nothing that needed to be cured.

But you keep reading: "Fortunately, most types of thyroid cancer have a very good prognosis when diagnosed early and treated by a physician who is familiar with its management."

Now the message is clear. The key to surviving thyroid cancer—that is, to having "a very good prognosis"—is early diagnosis and good medical care. And in case you're still missing the point, there is usually a patient's story to drive it home. And it goes something like this:[3]

It all began in 2008. Michelle was experiencing pain in her ear. While she was having it examined, the ENT doctor noticed a lump in her throat and, based on the blood work he did, recommended a biopsy.

"It was total luck that he noticed it, considering that the pain in my ear isn't typically a symptom for a thyroid problem nor did I have a particularly enlarged thyroid gland," Michelle said. "I decided to heed his advice."

Pain in the ear is not a symptom of a thyroid problem. Nevertheless, Michelle receives a neck exam to feel her thyroid. In other words, she was screened. And thyroid cancer was found. The story continues:

Even though it was an early cancer, Michelle was scared. So she called her mom in Philadelphia. "I figured my mom would know what to do next," Michelle recalled; she spent the week "in a blur." Her mother arranged for treatment at Fox Chase Cancer Center. In one five-hour surgery, her head and neck surgeon performed a thyroidectomy to completely remove her thyroid.

A month after the surgery, Michelle underwent radioactive iodine (RAI) therapy. After the RAI treatment, Michelle began taking a synthetic thyroid hormone to replace missing thyroid hormone and treat thyroid cancer.

"Stabilizing my thyroid was one of the more difficult aspects of this whole process since one's thyroid controls their metabolism.

"I now feel great."

Michelle ran her first triathlon, raising roughly $4,000 for the Leukemia and Lymphoma Society's event in September of 2006.

"I also volunteer to help women diagnosed with thyroid cancer," Michelle said. "Many people hear the 'C' word and start freaking out, without realizing how treatable the condition is. I share my experiences to give them strength."

Despite this compelling story, you actually have learned nothing about the value of looking for thyroid cancer early. You have learned something, though, about one person's experience with a side effect of undergoing treatment—it can be difficult to stabilize thyroid-replacement therapy after removing the thyroid. But there are no good hard facts here to guide your decision about whether to be screened for thyroid cancer.

Even without good facts, this Web site conveys a persuasive message: you should have your thyroid checked. And the words *thyroid cancer* can be replaced with any of a number of diseases to make the same basic argument—get checked to see if you have early disease; it's the "safe" thing to do.

But what if Michelle's cancer was not destined to progress? Then her surgery and subsequent treatment were all for nothing. When you acknowledge the very real possibility that you might be overdiagnosed, suddenly early detection doesn't sound so safe. There are a number of problems with this type of message. There is the failure to distinguish between an epidemic of disease and an epidemic of diagnosis. There is the assumption that patients who do well, do well because of treatment, not because they were going to do well anyway. And there is the use of a personal anecdote as a substitute for good hard facts.

The Web site of the American Society of Endocrinologists reports that thyroid cancer is one of the fastest-growing cancers in America. It's understandable that readers might assume that this means there is a true increase in the amount of disease: an epidemic of disease. But in fact, it more likely represents an epidemic of diagnosis. While it's true that there are a lot more people being told they have thyroid cancer now than there were in the past, that doesn't necessarily mean the burden of disease has changed, that more people have symptoms, complications, or are dying from thyroid cancer. It may instead reflect changing diagnostic practice: finding abnormalities that don't need to be found. (Ironically, the reason thyroid cancer is the fastest-growing cancer may be this organization's push for more screening!) Distinguishing an epidemic of disease from an epidemic of diagnosis is not something people can easily do on their own. But once you recognize that some epidemics are actually the result of medical care, you can at least pose a few questions. In the case of thyroid cancer, researchers have found that all the evidence points to an epidemic of diagnosis: a rapid rise in thyroid cancer diagnosis, but no increase in thyroid cancer death.

Doing well following early detection may say less about the value of early detection and more about the natural course of the kind of abnormality that can be detected early. It's great that most people with thyroid cancer have a very good prognosis. But just because people do well following early diagnosis and treatment doesn't necessarily mean they did well *because* of early diagnosis and treatment, as the Web site proclaims. Given the tremendous amount of overdiagnosis of thyroid cancer, many patients did well because they were going to do well anyway. Stating the favorable outcomes following early diagnosis is probably the most common tactic used in messages intended to persuade people to get checked. Often this tactic is buttressed by numbers: survival statistics. These are arguably the most misleading numbers in medicine.

Personal anecdotes are very effective motivators, but they say nothing about the value of early diagnosis and treatment. It's wonderful that Michelle did well. Everybody loves a story with a happy ending. People are engaged by all sorts of stories. Journalists are taught to begin some articles with a personal story. Consequently, personal stories appear all over the news and entertainment media. (I even included some in this book.) A story about a single named individual can be a great way to bring abstract ideas to life. But it is not the way to decide whether or not you will benefit from early diagnosis and treatment. A person whose life was apparently saved by screening might not have needed treatment in the first place, and a person who apparently died because he or she failed to get screened might have had an aggressive, untreatable cancer that couldn't have been detected early or that wouldn't have responded to treatment if it had been. Whether the personal anecdote is about a life saved because of screening or about a life lost because of screening's absence, the message is the same: screening is invaluable. Whenever you hear anecdotes like these, consider that there are alternative interpretations, those listed in table 10.1.

TABLE 10.1 *Two Generic Stories, Their Intended Messages, and Their Alternative Interpretations*

|  | **Good-outcome Story** | **Bad-outcome Story** |
|---|---|---|
| **Typical example** | Betty was screened and had her disease detected early. She is now well and is encouraging others to get screened. | Bill ignored recommendations to get screened. He now suffers with advanced disease (or has died) and he (or his family) regrets his decision. |
| **Intended message** | Those who pursue early detection can avoid the consequences of disease. Screening saves lives. Get screened. | All who suffer from disease could have avoided it had they sought early detection. Screening saves lives. Get screened. |
| **Alternative interpretations** | 1. Betty might not have needed to be diagnosed (i.e., she was overdiagnosed). | 1. Bill's disease might have been missed despite an early-detection effort. |
|  | 2. Betty would have done just as well if she had been diagnosed after developing symptoms (and would have avoided some time as a patient). | 2. Bill's disease might have been no more treatable even if it had been detected early. |
|  | 3. Betty's story is not over. She may yet die (or suffer) from her disease despite early detection and treatment. |  |

With all this in mind, you can imagine a different rendering of Michelle's story. (Note: All the quotations are from real patients' descriptions of their thyroid cancer treatment, posted on the Web.)

Michelle had ear pain. But instead of focusing on her primary complaint, her ENT doctor screened her for thyroid cancer. He thought he felt a lump in her neck.

Michelle was confused. She'd wanted help for her ear pain but was now being told she needed a thyroid biopsy. After he described the horrible consequences (and treatments) of advanced thyroid cancer, she felt she had to follow the doctor's advice.

Before she knew it, she'd undergone a five-hour surgery, during which a head and neck surgeon not only performed a thyroidectomy but also removed seventy-eight lymph nodes from her neck.

A month after the surgery, Michelle still had a sore neck and a weak voice. She was told that the surgery might not have completely removed her thyroid gland and that she needed radioactive iodine therapy to destroy any remaining thyroid tissue.

To prepare for the therapy she had to go on a two-week iodine-free diet, which meant no milk products. "Reading the diet makes me feel like I really can't eat anything." She was admitted to the hospital for the treatment itself, and the radiologist brought in an egg-shaped lead case with a vial containing one purple pill.

"He used forceps and transferred the pill into a small cup. He told me to pick up the cup and take the pill with lots of water. He evacuated the room rather fast after I took the pill. I guess he didn't want to get radiated. I guess I would do the same if I didn't have cancer to treat. After waiting about five minutes, the radiation officer approached the door and used a special device, a Geiger counter, to measure my radiation levels.

"For the next seven days I had to avoid people . . . my husband . . . my dog . . . pretty much everything."

She was given synthetic thyroid hormone because without her thyroid she could no longer make it herself.

At first, she lost weight. She noticed she was sweating more and that her heart raced. She told the doctors, who realized she was getting too much thyroid hormone. After the dose was decreased, she gained weight. Too much weight. And she was constipated and tired all the time. The doctors tried an intermediate dose.

"I now know that when I become hypothyroid [too little thyroid hormone] my system just shuts down. I become so lethargic that I can't even make it through half the day. Being hypothyroid was miserable and my heart goes out to anyone that can't get out of the hypothyroid state.

"Stabilizing my thyroid was one of the more difficult aspects of this whole process since one's thyroid controls their metabolism."

She developed a new interest in the politics of health care. "Now that I have a 'pre-existing condition' I am curious how this could affect my health coverage. I just finished watching President Obama's town-hall meeting about health-care reform. When he was talking about pre-existing conditions and health insurance companies denying coverage it really hit home for me. I wonder how this health-care reform will play out."

She read more about thyroid cancer and was surprised to find that many more people have thyroid cancer than ever die from it. She was particularly struck by the fact that despite all the additional thyroid cancers being found, the death rate from thyroid cancer remains unchanged.

Although her ear pain is long gone, she still suffers the side effects of her thyroid cancer treatment. She wonders if she should have taken the doctor's advice. She wonders if she went through all this for nothing. She wonders if she should see a lawyer, not a doctor.

Feels different, doesn't it?

### The common, but faulty, quantitative comparison

Numbers have a way of making things more persuasive. I think that's why some use the phrase *hard numbers*. But even hard numbers can be misleading. Imagine you are interested in learning the value of screening mammography in the elderly. You come across a news story entitled "Mammography May Be Beneficial to All Women, Regardless of Age."[4] In it, you find the following survival statistics:

> In women who are eighty years old or older, the five-year survival for breast cancer patients was 82 percent among those who did not use mammography and 94 percent among those who did.

Assuming the numbers are right (which they probably are), this statement seems to argue strongly that mammography is of value in the elderly. Only 82 percent of elderly women with breast cancer survive five years if they forgo mammography, while 94 percent survive five years if they undergo mammography. Seems clear-cut: mammography is the way to go. But, surprisingly, these numbers tell you nothing about the value of mammography in elderly women.

The statement is simply the numerical version of the generic message that there are favorable outcomes following early diagnosis. But when the numbers seem so compelling, it is even more difficult to see how those favorable outcomes might say less about the value of early detection and more about the natural course of the newly detected disease.

The most basic problem is that the data so often reported in news stories like the one above do not come from randomized trials. Rather, these data compare people who chose to be screened with people who chose not to be screened, and these groups may differ in many important ways other than the decision about mammography. In general, people who choose to be screened tend to be better educated, wealthier, and more attentive to their health overall (they are more likely to exercise and less likely to smoke, for instance). So while this kind of comparison is convenient, it is not fair. People who choose to be screened are bound to do better than others simply because they are healthier to start with, not because they are screened. (And note that this is about a lot more than being "health conscious"; it's about income and other socioeconomic factors that influence health.)

But even if these two groups of women were comparable in every way except the decision about mammography, even if this data had come from a randomized trial, the difference in their five-year survival still proves nothing about the value of mammography. Imagine that 1,000 women were diagnosed with breast cancer five years ago. If 820 are alive today, the five-year survival is 820/1,000, or 82 percent. If 940 are alive today, it is 940/1,000, or 94 percent. But even if screening mammography had raised the five-year survival from 82 percent to 94 percent, as the news story proclaims, it is entirely possible that no one who underwent screening lived even a day longer than she otherwise would have. This apparent paradox has two explanations, what epidemiologists call lead-time bias and overdiagnosis bias. Each is best understood by working through a simple thought experiment in which you begin by assuming that screening doesn't help anyone live longer and end by demonstrating how five-year survival can nevertheless increase.

*Lead-time bias*
Imagine a group of women with breast cancer who will all die of breast cancer at age ninety, whether they are diagnosed by mammography or by clinical symptoms. If they all receive the diagnosis at age eighty-six based on clinical symptoms, their five-year survival will be 0 percent. Because they all die at age ninety, each will live only four years from the time of diagnosis. Now imagine these same women had gotten mammography. Mammography finds cancers earlier; let's say two years earlier (that's the lead time). So now all of the women will be diagnosed at age eighty-four instead of eighty-six. All of a sudden, the five-year survival for these women will be 100 percent, even though they will all still die at age ninety. Earlier diagnosis *always* increases survival (in this case, five-year survival), but it doesn't necessarily prolong life. This effect is called lead-time bias and is illustrated in figure 10.1.

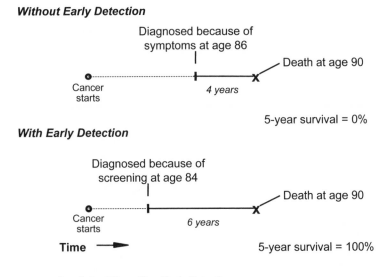

FIGURE 10.1 *Lead-time Bias—How Early Detection Can Increase Survival without Lengthening Life*

Of course, this is a simplification. I have supposed that all the women were diagnosed early, at age eighty-four. But not everyone has to be diagnosed early for this bias to take effect. All it takes is some people whose time of diagnosis is moved up to more than five years prior to death. Survival statistics will go up, even if no one's death is delayed. Making a diagnosis earlier will always increase survival from the time of diagnosis, but in this case, "increased survival" may simply mean that you know about your cancer for a longer time.

*Overdiagnosis bias*
Even if no lives are saved, survival statistics can also increase following early diagnosis if there is overdiagnosis. If early detection identifies abnormalities that meet the pathologic definition of cancer (that is, appear to be cancer under the microscope) but will never progress to cause symptoms or death, survival statistics will look more impressive. Imagine a city in which 1,000 women have symptoms of breast cancer—each feels a lump in her breast. Five years after diagnosis, 700 are alive and 300 have died. The five-year survival is 70 percent. Now let's turn back the clock and imagine that every woman in the city gets a screening mammogram. Now perhaps 1,500 would be given a cancer diagnosis: the 1,000 destined to develop lumps plus 500 others who are overdiagnosed. These 500 will not die from breast cancer in five years (because their cancer was never destined to progress). Nevertheless, the five-

### Without Early Detection

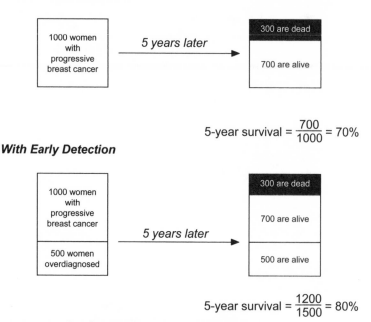

$$\text{5-year survival} = \frac{700}{1000} = 70\%$$

### With Early Detection

$$\text{5-year survival} = \frac{1200}{1500} = 80\%$$

FIGURE 10.2  *Overdiagnosis Bias—How Overdiagnosis Can Increase Survival without Saving Anyone's Life*

year survival for breast cancer in the city would increase to 80 percent; out of 1,500 women diagnosed, 1,200 of them will survive, including the 500 who have been overdiagnosed. But what has really changed? Five hundred people have been unnecessarily told they have cancer (and may have experienced the harms of therapy), but the number of deaths has not changed. Either way the same number of women, 300, have died from breast cancer. This effect is called overdiagnosis bias and is illustrated in figure 10.2.

Lead-time and overdiagnosis biases always combine to inflate survival statistics following early diagnosis. And the magnitude of their combined effect can be much larger than that illustrated here; instead of increasing survival statistics from 70 percent to 80 percent, these biases can increase the numbers from 5 percent to 90 percent. All it takes is a lot of lead time and a lot of overdiagnosis.

In both thought experiments, I made an assumption in order to simplify the numbers, namely, that there is no benefit (and no harm) from early diagnosis. But you should know that these biases occur regardless of the true effect of early diagnosis. If the true effect of early diagnosis really is some benefit, the biases will make that apparent effect larger. If the true effect is some harm (people's lives being shortened by unneeded treatment, for example), the biases will obscure that harm and can still make early diagnosis appear beneficial.[5]

Finally, it's important to point out that there's nothing special about the five-year interval. The two biases are equally relevant for any survival statistic measured from the time of diagnosis: two-year survival, ten-year survival, seven-and-a-half-year survival, and so on.[6]

### Randomized trials: The only source of unbiased data on the value of early detection

Because survival comparisons of diseases detected early versus those detected late are so biased, randomized trials measuring the rate of death are the only reliable way to get good hard facts about the value of early detection.

As you know, a randomized trial is a study in which enrolled patients are randomly assigned either to receive treatment or not. But for researchers to really learn something of value about early detection, there is a slight twist: the patients must be enrolled prior to being diagnosed. In a randomized trial of early detection, perfectly healthy people are randomly assigned to the look-early group or the control group. The expectation is that some people in the screening group will have the asymptomatic abnormality being sought and that they will then be treated. The trial is designed to compare how the look-early group does in relation to the group that is not screened.

Randomization prior to diagnosis is the best way to fully capture the effects of early detection. It is the way we studied screening mammography, fecal occult-blood tests for colon cancer, PSA screening for prostate cancer, and abdominal aortic aneurysm screening; it is the way we are currently studying spiral CT screening for lung cancer. The beauty of this design is that it specifically examines the effect of looking harder and answers a range of questions: Do people have a lower rate of death if they are screened? What other tests and procedures do they have to endure to determine if their early abnormality is a problem? What side effects or complications do they suffer relative to those who don't undergo screening? How many more people are diagnosed because of screening? (And, with longer follow-up, how many are overdiagnosed?)

The reality is that very few of the screening tests we do on asymptomatic individuals have been subjected to this standard. This includes routine physical examinations, routine blood tests, and imaging tests (such as total-body CT screening). And there are no randomized trials on the value of early detection for a variety of cancers, such as skin, bladder, kidney, pancreatic, ovarian, testicular, or thyroid cancer.

### See through exaggerated results—move beyond the relative frame

So imagine you have found a randomized trial of screening for abdominal aortic aneurysm in which randomization occurred prior to diagnosis. The media might report the results like this: "Screening for abdominal aortic aneurysm cut the death rate from rupture by almost half (44 percent)." Is that enough for you to assess the value of screening? That's a statement of relative risk, the kind you will often hear in the media. Cut in half sounds big. But if you know the underlying absolute risks—that the death rate has been reduced from 3.4 per 1,000 to 1.9 per 1,000 over five years—you are better positioned to judge the size of the effect. Regardless of what a person does, the chances of *not* having a ruptured aneurysm are greater than 996 per 1,000. But you can't possibly know that without seeing the numbers for absolute risk.

Relative risk tells you very little. One relative risk (say, reducing a risk by half) is compatible with an infinite number of absolute-risk pairs (from 500 to 250 per 1,000; from 100 to 50 per 1,000; from 20 to 10 per 1,000; from 4 to 2 per 1,000; from 0.1 to 0.05 per 1,000; and so on). The basic idea is fairly simple: reducing the risk of a common cause of death (one that affects 500 people out of 1,000, for instance) by 44 percent is more important than reducing the risk of a rare cause of death by 44 percent. Relative risk obscures this fact. But despite this weakness, the media makes a lot more announcements of relative risk than of absolute risk. The main reason, I think, is that relative changes generally look much more dramatic than absolute changes.[7] This is particularly true when the risk being reported is very small. Which sounds more impressive to you: reducing your risk by 44 percent or reducing it from 3.4 per 1,000 to 1.9 per 1,000? To persuade people to pursue early detection, relative risks are far more effective than absolute risks.

### Consider both sides of the story

Finally, it's not enough to know what the chances are that you'll be helped by early detection. You also need to know what the chances are that you won't be helped, that you'll be worried needlessly, that you'll be overdiagnosed and treated for no reason, or that you'll be hurt by treatment. A good randomized trial can provide all the information required to get the big picture (although it may not be easy to find all the information in one report).

To show you what I mean, let me return to the best-studied screening test: screening mammography. Worldwide, over a half a million women have been studied in ten randomized trials. The trials' findings aren't all the same, but the consensus is that mammography does help. Combining data from all the trials, the best estimate is that mammography reduces the death rate from breast cancer by about 20 percent.[8] That's a statement of relative risk. Here are the current absolute risks of breast cancer death for the typical fifty-year-old woman over the course of ten years: from about 5 per 1,000 without mammography to 4 per 1,000 with mammography. That means about 1,000 women have to be screened for ten years for one to benefit.[9]

While it's easy to focus on the one woman who benefits, what about the other 999? They get screened but do not benefit. For each woman who benefits, at least two are overdiagnosed and treated needlessly. Some have estimated the number to be as high as ten.[10] Furthermore some women, about 5 to 15 per 1,000, will have their cancer detected at a younger age with mammography, yet their prognosis will remain unchanged (those destined to die still will; those destined to survive would have done just as well if diagnosed later)—so they just live longer knowing they have cancer. And many women, 250 to 500 per 1,000, will experience a false alarm—a mammogram that indicates cancer might be present but that is ultimately proved wrong (by a second mammogram or a biopsy). This number is particularly high in the United States, where researchers have estimated that over a ten-year period, half the women who get annual mammography have at least one false alarm, and about a fifth of them have at least one biopsy.[11]

I think table 10.2 serves as a template for the kind of balanced information people need to make truly informed choices about whether or not to be screened.

TABLE 10.2  *Both Sides of the Story—A Balance Sheet*
*for Screening Mammography in Fifty-year-old Women*

| Among 1,000 fifty-year-old women undergoing annual mammography for ten years: | |
| --- | --- |
| Benefits | Harms |
| 1 will avoid a breast cancer death | 2 to 10 will be overdiagnosed and treated needlessly |
| | 5 to 15 will be told they have breast cancer earlier than they would have otherwise but this will have no effect on their prognosis[12] |
| | 250 to 500 will have at least one false alarm *(about half of these will be biopsied)* |

We aren't often presented with this balanced picture, but some are beginning to demand a complete accounting of the effects of early detection.[13] In the United Kingdom, researchers and patient advocates recently convinced the British National Health Service to rewrite their mammography screening pamphlets and explicitly lay out these numbers, giving patients accurate information about overdiagnosis for the first time.

■    ■    ■

SOME OF THE MOST COMPELLING health messages you will hear are about early detection of disease. Unfortunately, much of the evidence behind these messages is not so compelling. The benefits of early detection are often unknown but are bound to be small, simply because so few healthy people will develop the problem that it's attempting to fix. So good studies—randomized trials—have to involve a lot of people for a long period of time.

When those studies exist, remember that it's not enough to know that the test helped people. You want to know how much it helped people: how much the absolute risk of death (or advanced disease) was changed by early detection. You also want to know what people were put through to achieve this benefit: how many got tested, how many had false alarms, how many were overdiagnosed, and how many were harmed by unneeded treatment. These data are not as accessible as they ought to be. I hope they will be in the future (a number of researchers are working on this).

But the reality is that you will hear a lot of messages promoting the value of early detection when there have been no randomized trials to back up those claims. The messages will instead use convenient but faulty numbers (like five-year survival), tell personal anecdotes about people whose lives were "saved," or try to scare you by implying that a new epidemic is out there. None of this information tells you what you really want to know: does early detection lower the risk of death?

# CHAPTER 11

# Get the System

WHAT'S DRIVING OVERDIAGNOSIS? AT THE most basic level, it's driven by doctors' interest in making diagnoses. It's what we are trained to do: listen to patients, examine them, and test them to figure out what is wrong. Increasingly, however, we have also become concerned about what *may* go wrong in the future—that is, about making early diagnoses. That is what makes overdiagnosis possible. Overdiagnosis can occur only when people are given diagnoses and labeled as abnormal or at risk before they have symptoms.

But what's driving us to make more early diagnoses? If you have read any of the books criticizing the medical care system, it's easy to think that it's all about money, and that the number-one culprit is the pharmaceutical industry. More diagnoses mean more medicines are prescribed, generating more profit. If you ask a doctor what he or she thinks is driving early detection, the answer will typically include the word *lawyers* (along with a few choice adjectives). You might also hear the phrase *patient demand.* And if you were to talk to some in the public health community or to any number of organizations that advocate on behalf of patients with specific diseases, you would identify another plausible answer: true belief. Many genuinely believe that making more early diagnoses will help people live longer, happier lives. The truth is that all of these answers have some validity. In fact, there is a complex web of forces at work driving early detection and, consequently, overdiagnosis.

### Selling treatments for the well

Although I don't fly as much as many of my professional colleagues do (because the nearest real airport is an hour and a half from Dartmouth, and winter driving in northern New England is no fun), I do fly sometimes and I occasionally sit next to some interesting folks on the plane. Recently, I sat next to a pharmaceutical representative, a person who works as a member of the sales force for pharmaceutical companies. Because I work for the Department of Veterans Affairs, I rarely see drug reps in the workplace. The VA has stringent rules limiting the representatives' activities, and since the VA hospitals carry only a limited number of drugs anyway, they're not very good customers for the new, expensive drugs. The little contact I have had with drug reps, however, I have generally enjoyed. They are an interesting group. They tend to be smart. They are remarkably conversant in the biomedical science relevant to the drugs they represent and are highly skilled marketers. Part of their job is to engage in stimulating conversations with doctors. And they are very good at it.

At thirty thousand feet, this drug rep was telling me about a new drug called Forteo. It's a drug for osteoporosis, a condition that, he wanted to be sure I understood, had major public health implications. Millions of women have it (he might even have used the words *suffer from it*). Forteo is a synthesized portion of the naturally occurring parathyroid hormone, or PTH for short. PTH stimulates bone formation. So does Forteo. I was interested to learn all this. But I wanted to know if the drug really helped anybody. He told me about a randomized trial comparing the new drug to placebo in over sixteen hundred women[1] and the significant benefits found in terms of bone density, bone volume, and bone mass. He talked about how everyone in the study who had taken Forteo had had X-rays and bone-density scans that proved the bones were now more dense. But I still wanted to know whether the drug had helped anybody. The reason to treat osteoporosis isn't to make your bones look better on a scan (this doesn't necessarily make you feel or look any better). The only reason to treat osteoporosis is to reduce the number of bone fractures. He acknowledged that that was a good point. But he was ready for it. He communicated the data showing that the drug reduced the number of spinal compression factures.

How serious are compression fractures of the spine? It depends. A compression fracture is a narrowing of the height of an individual vertebra in the back. The vertebrae are like a stack of hollow bricks supporting the weight of the body. A compression fracture occurs when one of those bricks is compressed by that weight. The fractures sometimes hurt a great deal, but the majority are silent and don't hurt at all. Usually, the only way a person even knows she has one is if it is discovered by an X-ray. So does Forteo help reduce the number of fractures that actually bother people? Or does it simply reduce the ones people never would have known about if they hadn't been seen on X-rays?[2] In fact, the drug did appear to reduce the amount of "new or worsening back pain" from 23 percent to 17 percent over about two years.

But what I really wanted to know about was not compression fractures but hip fractures. There is no ambiguity with these fractures. They are never silent—they always matter. People with hip fractures can't walk. Virtually all require hospitalization. They need to have pins put in their hips or have their hips replaced entirely. And there's little doubt that having a hip fracture is a major risk factor for death. The drug rep said the study wasn't able to look at that. "But," he said, "there isn't a person on the planet who doesn't believe that this drug substantially reduces the risk of hip fracture."

I begged to differ. I told him he was sitting next to one. This got a good laugh. And his demeanor changed markedly. It turned out he was a pretty nice guy. He was interested to learn that there was a medical school filled with other doctors who might ask him similar questions. And then he let his guard down. "You know, if we really wanted to prevent hip fractures we'd take a different approach. Patients get hip fractures because they fall. Preventing falls in the elderly would go a longer way towards reducing hip fractures than all the medications in the world." I told you these guys were smart. But the bottom line is that drug reps are salespeople—men and women whose job is to help pharmaceutical companies make money, and pharmaceutical companies have a strong financial interest in pushing early treatment for all kinds of diseases.

Incidentally, the Forteo study was stopped early. It was supposed to be a three-year study, but it was stopped short of two years because rats in a long-term study of it developed bone cancer. While the FDA approved the drug, it required the company to conduct a ten-year trial looking for increased osteosarcoma in users of the drug (in the meantime, the FDA forbade the company to distribute free samples to physicians or to conduct direct-to-consumer advertising). Unfortunately, no results of the postmarketing surveillance were available nearly ten years later. As of this writing, Forteo is still on the market.

### Money

I don't think there's anything wrong with making money.[3] It's how our economy works. I'm glad the Apple computer company wants to make money. I use their products because I think they are superior (so much so that I even pay more for them). Owing to Apple's existence, PCs are better than they otherwise would be. We are getting these superior products *because* Apple wants to make money. I'm glad Priceline.com—the Web site that allows you to bid for travel services—wants to make money. I use their product because it helps me save money on car rentals (and because I'm glad to see William Shatner on TV again). Rental-car companies use Priceline for the simple reason that it helps them rent more cars. We are getting this more efficient market *because* Priceline wants to make money.

Unlike most of my medical-school classmates, I was not a biology or biochemistry major in college. I majored in economics. I was taught about the value of free markets—how they worked to create the goods and services people want in the right quantities and at the lowest possible prices. I also learned about the "invisible hand"[4]: how individuals pursuing their own self-interests—and their desire to make money—can improve the welfare of the larger society. But I do think that the drive to make more money has become a bad thing for medical care.

The problem is that medical care is nowhere close to being a free market. In a truly free market, called a *perfect market* in classic economics, buyers shop competitively and seek the best value, a trade-off between price and quality. But in medicine, few patients actually pay providers directly. Most are insulated from full price by having insurance. Patients rarely even know the prices of services; when they do find out, it's usually *after* they have received those services. Medical care violates a number of perfect-market conditions, shown below.

TABLE 11.1  *Perfect-market Prerequisites and the Realities of Medical Care That Violate Them*[5]

| Perfect-market Prerequisites | Medical Care Realities |
|---|---|
| Buyers pay full price. | Patients frequently insulated from price by insurance. |
| Buyers know the price. | Providers don't disclose price (*and may not even know it themselves*). |
| Buyers can make judgments about quality. | Patients largely don't know what services they need, what the options are, or what benefit they can reasonably expect. They need guidance from doctors about what services they should consume. |
| Buyers make rational decisions about price/quality options. | Sick and suffering patients are in a poor position to think rationally about options. And few people find it easy to think rationally when it comes to death. |
| Sellers unable to influence demand for their products. | Providers can create demand by telling patients what they "need." |

Perfect markets require, for instance, that buyers are able to judge quality. In the context of medical care, quality is an expansive concept—it's much broader than simply technical prowess (how quickly or safely a surgery is performed, for example). To judge the quality of medical care, buyers need to understand what they can expect without medical intervention, what the options are for intervention, and the likely benefits and harms (for instance, how strong the case is for a specific surgery). This isn't like the market for rental cars or computers, in which consumers largely understand the options available and know how much they value each of them. While it is possible (and in fact desirable) to inform patients about a few discrete decisions (like whether or not to have a hip replacement or whether or not to be screened), there's simply too much to know for consumers to be fully informed about all medical care consumption.

Perfect markets also assume that consumers' decision making will be rational, but that's a hard criterion to meet when patients are sick and suffering. Moreover, historically patients weren't given much of a chance to be involved in medical decisions. Under the traditional paternalistic model, doctors *ordered* things and patients *complied*. The change to a more participatory model (and the consumer movement in general) is a fairly recent development.

But the bottom line, the primary reason why medicine is nothing close to a perfect market, is that sellers in the medical care market are in an ideal position to create demand for their wares. How do they create demand? They decide that you need to consume their products. It's even embedded in the medical language: we write orders for consults, tests, or treatments. That's definitely not a characteristic of a perfect market. To be fair, the ability to create demand is not unique to medicine—the service department at my local Volvo dealer is fairly adept at it as well. But the problem is exacerbated in medicine because of the combined effect of the aforementioned factors: buyers' not paying the full price (or even knowing it); their having little idea about what medical care they need (or the benefits they can reasonably expect); and their being poorly positioned to think about options. Often patients don't have any way of knowing if treatments will help them or hurt them (so it's hard to judge their value). This is especially true for early diagnosis. People can't feel better after treatment when they weren't experiencing any symptoms to begin with. And no one can feel a change in the risk of having a bad outcome.

It is the perfect storm. Sellers create demand and exploit buyers to make more profit. And while it's always possible to sell more to those who are already buying, more treatments and more medicines, it's easier to increase sales by expanding the market to include new buyers. That is why more screening, turning more people into patients, is so great for business. Expanding the market for drugs has been a major driving force for redefining hypertension, diabetes, high cholesterol, and osteoporosis. Each of the consensus panels recommending these changes included individuals who had considerable financial ties to the sellers that were most likely to gain: the pharmaceutical companies.

The pharmaceutical industry has become the favorite whipping boy in discussions about the corrupting influence of money in medicine. And the companies deserve a lot of the criticism they receive. They are a problem, certainly, but I want to be clear that they are far from the *only* problem. The larger truth is that creating new patients and making more diagnoses benefits an entire medical-industrial complex that includes Pharma but also manufacturers of medical devices and diagnostic technologies, freestanding diagnostic centers, surgical centers, hospitals, and even academic medical centers.

Take screening, for instance. Screening can be a great loss leader for hospitals. A loss leader is an item a seller intentionally prices well below cost in an effort to stimulate other, profitable sales later. Supermarkets do this all the time. Increasingly, hospitals are trying it. The idea is simple: by offering screening at sharply reduced costs or, better yet, for free, hospitals are able to establish a new pool of patients and cash in on subsequent care. If you find this hard to believe, don't take my word for it—take Otis Brawley's. Dr. Brawley is an oncologist and epidemiologist and is now the chief medical officer for the American Cancer Society. Prior to that, he worked at the National Cancer Institute and was the director of the Georgia Cancer Center at Emory. While there, he made the following observation about "free" prostate cancer screening (Emory's loss leader) in a May 2003 interview with Maryann Napoli:[6]

> We at Emory have figured out that if we screen 1,000 men at the North Lake Mall this coming Saturday, we could bill Medicare and insurance companies for $4.9 million in health care costs [for biopsies, tests, prostatectomies, etc.]. But the real money comes later—from the medical care the wife will get in the next three years because Emory cares about her man, and from the money we get when he comes to Emory's emergency room when he gets chest pain because we screened him three years ago.
>
> . . . We don't screen anymore at Emory, once I became head of Cancer Control. It bothered me, though, that my P.R. and money people could tell me how much money we would make off screening, but nobody could tell me if we could save one life. As a matter of fact, we could have estimated how many men we would render impotent . . . but we didn't. It's a huge ethical issue.

He's right. It is a huge ethical issue. That's why I am so concerned about the corrupting influence of the commercialization of medicine.[7]

### True belief

People who want to make a profit drive the more-diagnosis movement for selfish reasons; true believers drive it for selfless ones. They sincerely believe that making more diagnoses is the path to better health for individuals and society. They see early diagnosis in particular as a cure-all. They believe it is the way to avoid advanced, symptomatic disease. And they envision a secondary gain from early diagnosis: avoiding the cost of treating advanced, symptomatic disease will save money for a cash-strapped system.

There are a lot of influential true believers: policy makers, politicians, members of the news and entertainment media, physician researchers, physician managers, and leaders of quality-improvement efforts and disease advocacy groups. A few of them largely understand the issues raised in this book. They fully understand the downside of overdiagnosis but tend to discount its human cost. Instead, they have a singular focus: do everything possible to avoid advanced disease, even if some will be harmed in the process. Most true believers simply don't question the conventional wisdom that early detection is always better. Many may have been swayed by personal experience. Physicians may feel that some of their patients' lives have been saved by screening, or they may be convinced that certain patients with advanced disease could have avoided their fates by early detection. Members of the general public may have similar views of their own experiences or of those of friends or family members. Some of these true believers may be vaguely aware of overdiagnosis but prefer to keep things simple and not have to deal with the nuances. Or they may not know about these issues and would be surprised to learn about them.

One of their beliefs that is clearly false is that early detection efforts will reliably save money. Because early detection always involves so many more people using medical care services, the strategy in fact tends to increase costs. More people are tested, more have abnormal tests (and surprise findings) that require more comprehensive testing, more then need follow-up visits, and more are eventually treated. As a result, any potential savings for the few who actually benefit from early detection are easily overwhelmed by the costs for the many who do not.[8]

### The resulting complex web

The convergence of the potential to generate a lot of profit with the efforts of true believers fuels a complex web promoting more diagnosis.

All of the major players—manufacturers, heath-care organizations, researchers, disease advocacy groups, and policy makers—are influenced by both financial gain and true belief, albeit to varying degrees. Manufacturers (those who make drugs or diagnostic and treatment devices) and health-care organizations (those who directly deliver these products) are largely influenced by the potential to profit. Simply stated, more diagnoses mean more patients for them and higher sales volumes. Nevertheless, they are undoubtedly also influenced by an element of true belief. Note that the combination is very powerful; it offers the prospect of "doing well by doing good."

Disease advocacy groups (for diabetes, thyroid cancer, and other disorders) and policy makers are largely composed of true believers. They promote more diagnosis because they believe it is the right thing to do for individuals and for society. Nonetheless, they also stand to profit from early diagnosis. Check out the Web site of any disease advocacy group and try to identify its major source of funds. Frequently, you will find that it is a manufacturer, usually a drug company, with a direct financial interest in treating the condition. Even policy makers are influenced by money, as the manufacturers and providers of medical care represent one of the largest sources of political donations, the third largest source, in fact.[9]

Researchers fall somewhere in the middle of this spectrum. Since I am one, I can tell you more about us. Researchers may or may not be true believers, but we are all influenced by money, specifically by grant money. The typical researcher is expected to obtain grants to fund specific research projects, funding that often subsidizes a substantial portion of his or her salary. While there are many sources of grant money, ranging from the federal government to pharmaceutical companies, there are always more researchers looking for money than there is money to be found. Putting together a grant is hard work. First, there's a lot of writing involved. This can be creative, but it's also terribly time consuming, and ironically it can distract from getting the actual research done. Then there is additional bureaucratic paperwork required: documents such as curriculum vitae, letters of support, institutional approvals, descriptions of research infrastructure, appendices detailing prior work, and so on. To be honest, I don't enjoy it very much.

And despite all this effort, most grant applicants don't receive funding. Consequently, researchers think hard about how to maximize their chances of persuading grant reviewers to fund their work. Reviewers are typically the most established researchers in their respective fields and many are wedded to conventional ideas and approaches—in fact, they may well have been the ones who established those conventions. So it's not surprising that researchers are typically cautious about proposing work that might discredit the conventional wisdom.[10] In this environment, a proposal to investigate ways to increase access to early detection is a fairly safe bet. (Some of us used to joke that any proposal to increase the use of mammography could get funded, even if it involved scaring women to persuade them to get screened.) A proposal to study early detection's side effects, however, is far less likely to receive funding. To be fair, this is changing to some degree. Some funding agencies, particularly those within the federal government, are now more open to grant proposals addressing some of the issues surrounding overdiagnosis. But the "better safe than sorry" dictum still persists.

The major players have many means to influence those they are trying to persuade of the need for more diagnosis, namely, members of the general public and the front-line doctors who serve them. The most obvious of these means is advertising. The United States is one of only two countries in the world that allow direct-to-consumer advertising of prescription drugs (the other is New Zealand).[11] Expenditures for direct-to-consumer drug advertising have grown explosively over the past fifteen years (if you watch much TV, this is something I'm sure you are painfully aware of); it's gone from just a few million dollars in 1990 (before the FDA provided guidance on what was acceptable television advertisement) to well over five billion dollars in 2006.

But the drug companies are not the only ones advertising. Increasingly, health-care organizations are too. It's hard to drive through an American city now without seeing at least one billboard for every local hospital. And it's not just hospitals; outpatient clinics, doctors, freestanding diagnostic centers, and academic medical centers all advertise. And many of these ads promote testing for early diagnosis.

Disease-awareness campaigns are a special form of advertising. Historically, these campaigns were conducted through public service announcements—that is, free advertising (the anti-smoking campaigns to reduce lung cancer, for example). That still happens, but increasingly, awareness campaigns involve paid advertising. And also increasingly, instead of promoting healthy lifestyles, the campaigns are pushing the early detection of disease, encouraging you to get checked for any one of a number of health concerns. Their funding sources reflect this: many are financed, directly or indirectly, by manufacturers or providers of drugs and screening devices.

Although advertising and disease-awareness campaigns exert their greatest influence on the general public, they influence doctors as well. But doctors are also influenced by the scientific literature, which, in turn, can be influenced by manufacturers who fund research. Most medical research is now funded by industry.[12] Industry strongly determines what research questions get pursued (which explains why there are far more studies on drugs to treat osteoporosis than on how to prevent the elderly from falling). And doctors can also be swayed by government reports, which are arguably the least biased sources of information.

And then there's the media. News and infotainment (such as talk shows) are always looking for engaging, simple stories. Stories about new diagnostic technologies or the value of early diagnosis fit the bill perfectly. Providers, researchers, and disease advocacy groups know this and are happy to supply the material. Unfortunately, these stories usually include a powerful but misleading anecdote—preferably a testimonial from a celebrity or a politician—and fail to include any discussion of the nuances involved in early detection. That, in a nutshell, is the system that promotes more diagnosis.

### People caught in the web

This complex web ultimately snares the general public; people hear the resounding messages that (1) you should be afraid about your health, and (2) the right response is to get checked. Most Americans believe that more diagnosis is in their interest, that it is the best strategy for good health, and that it is the safest thing to do.

The perceived value of more diagnosis is particularly strong for conditions that can be plausibly labeled *silent killers,* conditions people don't even know they have because they don't have any symptoms. The public has been taught to be particularly enthusiastic about early diagnosis, so searching for silent conditions is generally viewed as socially responsible. But as you know, this search is also something else: the prerequisite for overdiagnosis. You might hope that your doctor would serve as a counterbalance to all the forces promoting more diagnosis, but she is probably caught in the web too.

### Doctors inside the web

Some doctors do stand to profit greatly from more diagnosis. Doctors who have financial incentives to pursue more diagnosis include those who primarily do diagnostic procedures (such as gastroenterologists who do endoscopies and cardiologists who do heart catheterizations) and those who own testing equipment (such as radiologists who own imaging centers and primary care physicians who own the equipment to perform lab tests, stress tests, echocardiograms, and bone-density tests). For many doctors, however, the financial incentive is minute, if it exists at all.

And while some doctors are true believers, many wonder whether the use of diagnostic tests has pushed the boundaries of common sense. Some know full well that there are two sides to early diagnosis. So, many front-line docs, those engaged in the direct care of people who are candidates for more diagnosis, aren't blindly devoted to the concept of early diagnosis and don't stand to gain financially in this arena. They make very pragmatic, totally understandable (however undesirable) calculations about whether or not to pursue more diagnosis. An obvious consideration is the path of least resistance. Front-line docs are busy people. Ordering a test is both quick and simple; discussing with a patient why testing might not be in his or her interest is neither. It takes time and requires explaining the problem of overdiagnosis. Physicians' working assumption is that most people like being tested (it's a concrete service) and that very few object to it.

Another consideration for doctors in ordering tests may be less familiar to the public: our desire to get a good grade. Health-care organizations—hospitals, clinics, and so forth—have an increasingly strong interest in measuring the quality of medical care. Conceptually the idea is most laudable, but as is so often the case, the devil is in the details. Truly measuring the quality of care for sick patients is a real challenge. It requires detailed knowledge not only about the patient's disease but also about what other diseases he may have and what he wants out of his care. It means that we have to know what constitutes high-quality care in that particular setting. Consequently, we are struggling with this measurement problem. In contrast, counting how many people get a specific immunization or screening test is easy (whether or not this is really a meaningful measure of quality is another story). That's why preventive services were the original focus of health-care report cards—the measures of doctors and hospitals you might find on the Internet—with mammography being one of the most prominent. We doctors were selected by medical schools for our desire to get good grades. If ordering more screening tests leads to better grades, we'll do it.

Finally, there is the consideration of "safety first." We doctors like lawyer jokes. (My personal favorite: What do you have when two lawyers are buried up to their necks in sand? Not enough sand.) But the truth is that doctors are afraid of lawyers. Even though I suspect the perceived risk of malpractice suits is much larger than the real risk, all that matters here is the perception. We see that there are legal penalties for underdiagnosis (failure to diagnose) and no corresponding penalties for overdiagnosis. Deciding which is the "safer" strategy on that basis is not very challenging.

### Your doctor's nightmare

If doctors had to choose the most powerful incentive for pursuing more diagnosis, most of them would probably pick the one involving lawyers. The prospect of being sued is truly frightening. About a decade ago, a close friend of mine was taken to court for failure to diagnose prostate cancer. Joel was sued by a middle-aged man who had seen him twice for routine checkups. Joel had asked him if he had any complaints. He said he was fine. Joel checked his blood pressure and listened to his lungs. Both were normal. He did a rectal exam to feel both the prostate and the wall of the rectum (another potential cancer site). As is the case with many middle-aged men, this patient had a prostate that was enlarged but otherwise normal. On the first visit Joel also referred him for a sigmoidoscopy, one of the screening tests for colorectal cancer. It was normal too.

Six months later the patient started having trouble urinating. When he went to the bathroom he found it very hard to start a stream of urine. He saw a urologist, who repeated the rectal exam and felt the prostate. Now there was a growth. The urologist did a PSA; it was sky-high, suggesting that the patient had a cancer that had spread beyond the prostate. The urologist learned about the patient's previous visit with Joel and told him, "If your doctor had done a PSA six months ago, he would have saved your life."

At the risk of sounding like a stereotypic doctor defending the interests of his friend and profession, this is an egregious statement. Let's parse it out. Most important, at the time the diagnosis was made, there was no evidence that the PSA could save anyone's life. No one should suggest that someone's life would have been saved without some evidence that the strategy of early detection actually works. But even if PSA had been shown to detect some prostate cancers early enough to save some lives, the statement would still be egregious. It's far too definitive. If PSA worked, it is possible that it could have detected a deadly cancer six months earlier while it was more treatable. But it is also possible that it would not have made any difference for this particular patient. The cancer might not have been present six months earlier and therefore would not have been detected by any test, as is the case with many fast-growing, aggressive cancers. Or the cancer might have been detectable at the earlier visit but no more treatable, as is also typically the case for very aggressive cancers. Some cancers are very resistant to therapy; some metastasize early in their course; and others are simply not amenable to therapy (they are so close to vital structures that they cannot be removed without killing the patient).

Without a doubt, this patient had developed a very aggressive cancer. That's a terrible thing. Joel felt bad for him. All of us would have; something very unfortunate had happened to another human being. But the urologist compounded the tragedy by playing into an increasingly destructive (and common) mind-set in our society: something bad has happened, and thus someone must be at fault.

The case went to trial in a small town in Vermont. Experts on prostate cancer screening from the University of Connecticut and Harvard testified about what we knew at the time: that overdiagnosis was a real problem and that the benefit of PSA was unknown. But the local urologist told the jury an emotional story: This doctor failed to diagnose a deadly cancer. Add to that a real patient with advanced cancer, looking all the worse since he was suffering from the side effects of treatment. There were even courtroom theatrics. At one point, the patient's wife stood up, pointed at Joel, and yelled, "Murderer." I presume she was coached to do so, as Joel was coached to bring his wife and daughter to court to help humanize him.

You can probably guess the rest of the story. The jury found for the plaintiff. Joel's lawyers felt certain a more rational verdict could be obtained on appeal but that the cost of the process would likely exceed the proposed award. The verdict was accepted; the award was paid. Not surprisingly, Joel started ordering more PSAs. (There is some research showing that a doctor's being sued for failure to diagnose prostate cancer leads not only the defendant to order more PSAs but also his or her colleagues.[13]) He refers more patients to urologists, and they find more prostate cancer. While some of those patients may be helped, many more suffer the side effects of unneeded therapy.

I think the experience has had a more global effect on Joel. He doesn't want to be in a courtroom again. He doesn't want to be accused of failing to order a test. I think he orders more tests in general now. It makes sense. I don't know of any doctor who has had to appear in court because he or she *did* order a test. There are a lot of good doctors out there, doctors who would like to do the right thing, but anecdotes like this can drive the behavior of even the best of them. Doctors like to blame lawyers for excessive diagnostic testing. It is time to take this excuse off the table.

If policy makers really want to combat overdiagnosis, they are going to have to deal with the problem of asymmetric legal risks, of underdiagnosis being subject to penalty while overdiagnosis is not. While "failure to diagnose" is a perfectly legitimate suit against a doctor who saw a patient with symptoms of disease, it ought to be thrown out when brought on behalf of a patient who has the disease now but had no symptoms of disease at the time he or she was seen. All patients who have experienced dreaded health outcomes are asymptomatic for some period in their disease courses, and most have seen doctors during those long periods. So if "failure to diagnose" applies in this period, then virtually all physicians could be subject to this charge. For many conditions, we simply have no evidence that screening reduces anyone's chance of developing advanced disease, and even when we do have evidence that screening helps *some* people, it does not help those with fast-growing, aggressive cancers that are not detectable at the time of screening or that are resistant to treatment.

So even with good screening tests, people who are screened can still die from cancer. In fact, the typical plaintiff's argument is more likely to be wrong than right. Even in the case of mammography—the best-studied screening test—a plaintiff dying from metastatic breast cancer who made the typical argument that screening would have helped would be correct only one in five times.[14] Doctors' fear of malpractice shouldn't be the reason healthy people are subjected to more testing. The reason should be that people choose to undergo screening after being informed about the potential benefits and harms. Doctors should be held accountable for informing patients about proven early detection options but not for underdiagnosing patients who present with no symptoms.

### *The final wild card: intolerance of uncertainty*

I have covered the cultural forces that drive overdiagnosis, but there is one additional motive that leads us to stumble onto abnormalities. Often, doctors pursue aggressive testing in people who have vague symptoms that don't seem to indicate consequential disease. Fear of malpractice drives some of this testing, certainly, but it is not the main motivator. Instead, a lot of it has to do with an intolerance of uncertainty. The hope is that through diagnostic testing we will provide certainty that nothing is wrong, reassuring the patients (and ourselves).

Unfortunately, it may do neither. It may lead to more uncertainty and more anxiety. Just ask Michael. He's a reporter for a national men's magazine who called me to talk about prostate cancer screening but then related a story about a diagnosis that had nothing to do with prostate cancer (at least initially). Michael is a fundamentally healthy male in his forties. He went to his doctor because he noticed some pain on the right side of his back. But he wasn't sick; he didn't have a fever, a cough, trouble breathing, or any change in appetite. He had nothing other than pain, and that only when he took a deep breath, coughed, or lay down on his right side.

This sounds like pleurisy, an inflammation of the lining of the lung. For years we have known that in young, healthy people, it is most commonly the result of a viral infection. In the past, most doctors would have just made this presumptive diagnosis and reassured the patient that it would soon go away.

The pain did soon go away. Michael felt well the next day. But his doctor had ordered a chest X-ray. And the radiologist said that the X-ray showed signs of pneumonia. Michael's doctor was incredulous. Michael had no symptoms of pneumonia: he had no fever, no cough, no shortness of breath. The doctor ordered a CT scan of Michael's chest. Once again the radiologist found evidence of pneumonia, and once again, Michael's doctor wasn't buying it. He asked the radiologist to review the scan one more time.

On further inspection, the radiologist found a tiny blood clot in one of the small branches of the right pulmonary artery, one of arteries that supply the lung. It may or may not have caused his symptoms, which were now gone. Nevertheless, a blood clot in the lung gets doctors' attention. Michael was immediately started on heparin, a medication to keep blood from clotting (making bleeding much more likely). He was put in an ambulance, placed on a heart monitor, given oxygen, and rushed to the hospital.

Michael was getting scared. He was admitted to the hospital, but the doctors there couldn't find any obvious reason for him to have a clot. They did mention that people sometimes get clots when they have hidden cancers. Now Michael felt even worse.

Michael had all sorts of tests to look for cancer—blood tests, scans, and a colonoscopy. While waiting for the test results in his hospital bed, he fell prey to his catastrophic thinking. He started playing out all kinds of worst-case scenarios in his head: *What if cancer caused my clot? Am I dying? What will happen to my wife and kids?*

Michael grew increasingly anxious about the prospect of cancer, but none was found. However, he did have a follow-up appointment with a hematologist. The hematologist recommended that he stay on blood thinners for life. He would always face a higher risk of bleeding, but the blood thinners would prevent future clots. I'm happy to report that the story doesn't end there. A wise pulmonologist thought the whole thing was crazy. He told Michael that today's sophisticated scanning machines would pick up small clots in the lungs of many healthy people. This particular clot just happened to be in a spot where it temporarily irritated the pleural lining of the lung. He thought that Michael's risk of having a dangerous blood clot was extraordinarily low and that the suggestion of a lifelong blood thinner was drastic. He told Michael to stop the blood thinner and get on with his life.

Michael did that and feels fine physically. But even though he knows he is at average risk for cancer (maybe less, since he has a limited family history of the disease), he is still haunted by the idea that he might have cancer. He wakes up at night thinking about it. In effect, he's developed a cancer phobia due to the whole incident, severe enough that he had to see a psychologist. Michael believes, and so do his doctors, that this anxiety led to his new diagnosis: chronic pelvic pain syndrome—chronic tension in his pelvic-floor muscles leading to pain in the pelvis, groin, and genitals and to urinary symptoms of prostatitis (despite the absence of prostate infection or inflammation). It can be a debilitating problem. And given the location of the pain and the prostatitis symptoms, he's now worried about prostate cancer.

So a tiny blood clot in the lung, one that produced symptoms for only one day, has resulted in a cancer phobia. The anxiety, in turn, has produced chronic pelvic pain. And the associated symptoms have raised Michael's concern that he might have prostate cancer. He often wonders if he would have been better off if he had never seen a doctor.

The pursuit of diagnostic certainty can have real consequences. I have thought about this story a lot since Michael told it to me. Where did we go wrong? Why was the CT scan ordered? Why didn't the doctor stop, given that his patient was well? Maybe he was afraid of lawyers, but I doubt it. Why didn't the radiologist stop? Maybe she owned the CT scanner and wanted the income, but I doubt it. Instead, I suspect both wanted to do the best they could to pin down exactly what was going on. They thought they were providing Michael the best care possible. But they didn't consider that there might be downsides to pursuing diagnostic certainty. They didn't consider the problem of overdiagnosis.

# CHAPTER 12

# Get the Big Picture

NOW YOU HAVE A SENSE of the breadth of the problem of overdiagnosis. You know it can occur in a wide variety of conditions: from numerical abnormalities (like high blood pressure and high cholesterol) to structural abnormalities (be they in your knee or in your baby) to the most feared abnormality of all, cancer. You know that it is the result of many different mechanisms: looking harder for things to be wrong through more screening, expanding definitions of who is sick by altering the threshold for abnormal, and increasing the chance that we stumble onto something wrong by doing more diagnostic tests in general. You know how easy it is to be misled, by both stories and numbers, into thinking early diagnosis is always in your interest. And you know that the combined effect of the desire to make money and true belief has produced a medical culture that will not be easily dissuaded from the idea that earlier diagnosis is always better. I want to return here to the big picture to help you consider whether earlier diagnosis is really worth it.

*Morning rounds*

Most physicians begin their days by making rounds, the process of reviewing the cases and progress of their patients in the hospital. And I think reviewing the cases of the patients you have met in this book is a useful place for us to begin to see the big picture of overdiagnosis. So take a few minutes now and make rounds by perusing table 12.1, which provides a capsule review for each patient.

The worthy motivation for more and earlier diagnosis is to help people avoid the bad consequences of advanced disease. In a perfect world, diagnosis would lead only to benefit: fewer symptoms, fewer hospitalizations, and longer, healthier lives. But in the real world, diagnosis also has harms. While stories about lives saved from diagnosis are common, stories about people hurt by diagnosis are extremely rare. But people do get hurt all the time. Some of the harms are minimal, but some are quite severe. That is why I wanted to share the stories of these patients.

TABLE 12.1 *Summary of Possible Benefits and Harms Experienced by Patients in This Book*

| Patient | Condition Diagnosed | Possible Benefit |
|---|---|---|
| *Mr. Lemay* Fifty-seven-year-old with chest pain (chapter 1) | Severe hypertension | *Dramatically reduced chance* of something bad (stroke, heart attack, or death) happening over the next five years: 80% down to 8% |
| *Mr. Bailey* Eighty-two-year-old Vermont farmer (chapter 1) | Mild hypertension | *Reduced chance* of something bad (stroke, heart attack, or death) happening over the next five years: 18% down to 13% |
| *Mr. Roberts* Seventy-four-year-old with well-managed ulcerative colitis (chapter 2) | Mild diabetes | *Reduced chance* of diabetes complications |
| *Lara* Sixty-five-year-old New Yorker who summers in Vermont (chapter 2) | Osteopenia Possible thyroid cancer | None known |
| *Isaac* Fifty-year-old oncologist researcher (chapter 4) | Early prostate cancer found by PSA screening | None to at most a small *reduced chance* of dying from prostate cancer (about 1 man benefits per 1,000 screened) |
| *Mr. Baker* Sixty-year-old with hoarseness (chapter 7) | Incidentally detected kidney cancer | None known |
| *Natalie Angier* Pregnant *New York Times* science reporter (chapter 8) | Baby with a clubfoot | None known |
| *Ms. Smith* Hypothetical twenty-year-old undergoing baseline genome scan (chapter 9) | Various "risks" of future disease | None known |
| *Michael* Reporter for men's magazine (chapter 11) | Blood clot in lung | *Reduced chance* of subsequent clot |

| Chance That the Patient Was Overdiagnosed | Harm Experienced |
|---|---|
| **Zero** (he had symptoms from the condition) | *Minimal:* hassle factors associated with treatment |
| **Moderate** | *Moderate:* fainted because medication made his blood pressure too low |
| **Almost Certain** (he has not been treated since and has never experienced symptoms) | *Severe:* broke his neck because he fainted while driving when his medication made his blood sugar too low |
| **High** | *Moderate:* medication-induced esophagitis and rash, anxiety of possibly having thyroid cancer, associated testing and follow-up |
| **High** (fifty times more likely than being the one man who benefits) | *Moderate:* fatigue interfering with work for six weeks<br>*Severe:* impotence |
| **Certain** (never treated nor had symptoms, died from other causes) | *Moderate:* diagnosis of kidney cancer and associated testing, follow-up, and anxiety (Note: Harm could have been severe had he had the unneeded surgery—kidney failure, dialysis, and even death.) |
| **Certain** (baby did not have clubfoot) | *Severe:* severe anxiety and emotional distress for half of pregnancy |
| **High** | *Unknown:* anxiety about future, subsequent testing, possible intervention |
| **High** | *Moderate:* subsequent testing and treatment<br>*Severe:* anxiety about cancer |

The harms of diagnosis fall into three general categories. First, all patients experience the impact of the diagnosis itself. Being given the label of a diagnosis can make a person feel more vulnerable—it makes him think something is wrong, something he needs to worry about. Just ask Lara, Ms. Angier, or Michael. This induced vulnerability undermines the sense of well-being and resilience that in many ways defines health itself. So, ironically, the drive toward more and earlier diagnosis can conflict with the goal of a healthier society. And if you don't care about the psychological harm patients sustain, or if you believe it is a small price to pay to detect diseases early, consider the more practical harm in our health-care system: a diagnosis has made obtaining health insurance harder and more expensive. Worse, for some it has led to the loss of insurance altogether.

Second, most patients experience the impact of subsequent intervention, either treatment or more diagnostic evaluation. These are associated with numerous hassles: more phone calls, appointments, medication adjustments, more testing, more surveillance, more prescriptions, and so on. Lara, Mr. Baker, and Michael had to deal with many of these hassles. I think most would agree these inconveniences could also be characterized as harms.

Yet it is the third type of harm that is most consequential: some people experience adverse effects from the interventions that stem from diagnosis. Adverse effects may be transient (Mr. Bailey's fainting spell or Lara's esophagitis, for example), prolonged (Mr. Roberts's broken neck), or permanent (Isaac's impotence). They may range from mild medication side effects, to surgical complications, to problems requiring hospitalization, and even to death.

Diagnosis is only worth it if its benefits outweigh its harms. The potential benefit of diagnosis is directly related to the spectrum of the abnormality; in other words, to the severity of the condition being diagnosed. You might be wondering why I use the phrase *potential benefit* instead of simply the word *benefit*. The reason is that the actual benefit is related not only to the spectrum of the abnormality but also to how well treatment works. While the potential benefit may be very high, if treatment doesn't work well, the actual benefit will be very small.

Clearly there is no potential benefit in diagnosing and treating someone with a mild abnormality who is destined to stay healthy, and it is equally obvious that there is a great deal of potential benefit in treating someone who has a severe abnormality that can quickly lead to death. The potential benefit is intermediate for those whose abnormalities are in between. As you know, mildly elevated blood pressure is much less likely to lead to a heart attack or stroke than very high blood pressure is, so the potential benefit of diagnosis and treatment is much smaller for a patient like Mr. Bailey (who had mild systolic hypertension) than for a patient like Mr. Lemay (who came to the hospital with chest pain and very high blood pressure). But the relationship between the spectrum of the abnormality and the potential benefit of diagnosis is not limited to high blood pressure. This simple relationship applies to virtually all medical conditions. And since, with the exception of Mr. Lemay, all of the patients in our morning rounds have mild abnormalities, the potential benefit of diagnosis and treatment for each is necessarily small (if it exists at all).

And what about harms? They are always there, sometimes trivial, sometimes profound, but always much less consistently related to the spectrum of abnormality than benefits are. The anxiety related to diagnosis is probably influenced more by the label itself (being told one has cancer, for example) and by the individual's reaction to that label than by where the condition sits on the spectrum. Similarly, the hassle factors of subsequent follow-up and treatment are relatively independent of the spectrum and more related to the recommended therapies and the system delivering them. The relationship between the spectrum of the abnormality and the third category of harm—adverse effects from intervention—is more variable. Harms may be more likely when abnormalities are severe. The chances of having a surgical complication, for instance, are generally higher for an individual with a more severe abnormality, because the surgery involved is more complicated and there is more that can go wrong. But in conditions defined by numbers, such as hypertension and diabetes, the chance of harm from the side effects of medication may well be higher for individuals with milder abnormalities. People like Mr. Bailey are more likely to pass out from treatment-induced low blood pressure than people like Mr. Lemay. The reason is simple: Mr. Bailey's blood pressure was relatively low to begin with, while Mr. Lemay's blood pressure was so high that medication was unlikely to lower his blood pressure too much.

So the bottom line is that, while the potential benefit of diagnosis and treatment is strongly related to the spectrum of the abnormality, the harms of diagnosis and treatment are much less so. Figure 12.1 illustrates these relationships: a steeply rising line for potential benefit as abnormalities become more severe, and a flat line for harms (since it could arguably have a slightly positive slope, a slightly negative slope, or a slope anywhere in between).[1]

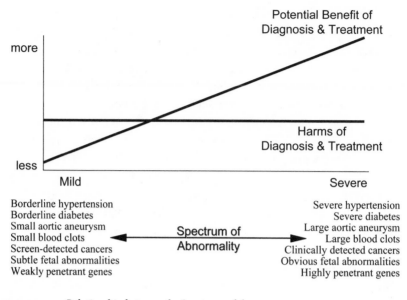

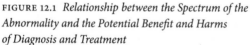

FIGURE 12.1 *Relationship between the Spectrum of the Abnormality and the Potential Benefit and Harms of Diagnosis and Treatment*

In theory, a simple calculation would allow us to assess the net effect of diagnosis: net effect = benefit − harm. But in practice, there's much more complexity. There's the problem that if treatment is ineffective, the actual benefit may be much smaller than the potential benefit. Then there's the problem that reliable numbers about the benefits and harms are often not available. And there's the apples-and-oranges problem: it's difficult to weigh benefits and harms when they are so dissimilar (for example, how many extra appointments and fainting spells would you accept to experience a small reduction in your chance of having a heart attack?). But don't let this complexity distract you from a pretty clear guiding principle. The people most likely to experience net benefit are those with the most severe abnormalities. Conversely, the people most likely to experience net harm are those with the mildest abnormalities. This principle is illustrated by the shaded areas in between the lines in figure 12.2.

Simple concept. Severe abnormalities warrant action because net benefit is likely. But the best strategy for mild ones may be to leave well enough alone, otherwise net harm is likely. In fact, it may be better not to look for them in the first place.

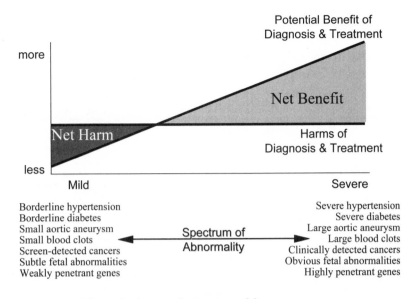

FIGURE 12.2  *Relationship between the Spectrum of the*
*Abnormality and the Net Effect of Diagnosis and Treatment*

### *How the search for mild abnormalities begins—*
### *the problem of excessive extrapolation*

You might think that all doctors would understand this trade-off, but they don't. Despite the subtleties and balancing acts involved in early diagnosis, most efforts to expand diagnoses to include milder abnormalities are not very controversial in the medical community. In fact, typically they are embraced. The rationale behind making more diagnoses works something like this: First, medical science identifies that some intervention improves an important health outcome in a high-risk group. Then someone makes the following supposition: what's good for a group on the severe side of the spectrum of abnormality (the high-risk group) is probably good for a group on the mild side of the spectrum of abnormality (the low-risk group). This is a problem of excessive extrapolation.

The issue with extrapolating from severe to mild abnormalities is that, practically speaking, it is often not known whether the same important benefits of treatment will appear in people with mild abnormalities. By *important benefits* I mean avoiding death or major complications of disease (such as a hip fracture or an advanced cancer). These events are so rare in those with mild abnormalities that it would require enormous studies to learn if treatment actually has an important benefit for this group. The studies required may need to be larger than any we could reasonably expect to conduct.[2] So investigators focus on less important but more measurable outcomes—such as bone density or PSA level—as surrogates. Even outcomes that seem important on initial inspection may be more ambiguous in reality: compression fractures of the spine (which patients may or may not feel) or the development of small cancers (which may or may not grow). Benefits in these surrogate and ambiguous outcomes may be demonstrable, but improvements in them do not reliably translate into improvements that matter, namely, whether people feel better or live longer. Instead they require a leap of faith, an inference that proof of measurable benefits portends the existence of important benefits. But real benefits are, at best, small and uncertain, and they can easily be overwhelmed by the associated harms of diagnosis, hassle factors, and adverse effects from intervention (although these harms typically are not even considered, much less measured).

Once someone decides that what is good for a high-risk group must be good for a low-risk group, the stage is set for more diagnosis. If doctors take up the call, as they generally have, the stage is also set for more harm. Because more diagnosis always means that we are diagnosing people with milder abnormalities, those that are less likely to lead to symptoms or to result in death, many patients are overdiagnosed. And since we don't know who has been overdiagnosed and who hasn't, we tend to treat everybody. Those who have been overdiagnosed cannot benefit from treatment; they can only be harmed. So "new" patients identified by more diagnosis are much more likely to experience net harm compared with patients diagnosed in the past.

More diagnosis triggers a self-reinforcing cycle, one that prompts doctors to diagnose more. In other words, it's a positive-feedback loop,[3] a cycle in which some effect causes more of itself, expanding and promoting that initial effect. Figure 12.3 shows how more diagnosis begets more diagnosis. Here's how it works. Someone somewhere makes an excessive extrapolation and suggests something that leads to more diagnosis; perhaps that something is more screening, or an expanded definition of abnormal, or more testing in general. Immediately, doctors notice that there are more abnormalities out there than they had previously thought, which in itself promotes more diagnosis. Then population-based health statistics, which reflect how many people have the disease (prevalence) or how many are newly diagnosed (incidence), appear to rise. Now the population appears sicker than previously thought. Someone uses the word *epidemic*. To make sure no cases are missed,

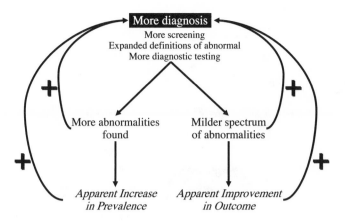

FIGURE 12.3  *The Self-reinforcing Cycle That Prompts Doctors to Pursue More Diagnosis*

more diagnosis is recommended. At the same time, the spectrum of detected abnormalities shifts toward milder forms. Doctors notice this as well. They see that the typical "patient" has milder disease than in the past and tends to do better. That in itself is seen as an accomplishment—an effect of better medical care—thereby promoting more diagnosis. Then diseased-based health statistics (such as measurements of five-year survival) appear to improve. Someone uses the phrase *save lives.* To "save" more lives, more diagnosis is recommended.

### *The self-reinforcing cycle for the public*

More diagnosis, the resulting "epidemics," and claims that testing that can save lives make the public want to seek more diagnosis as well. The public has been primed for this response, having been bombarded with messages about the value of getting tested from doctors, public health officials, the media, and maybe even their own mothers. People have not been encouraged to approach these messages critically, nor have they been taught how to judge whether these messages reflect solid science or are really just propaganda. But surprisingly, as the public gets more and more testing, the test results themselves promote more testing. It's a second self-reinforcing cycle, shown in figure 12.4. It works regardless of whether the test results are normal or abnormal. And it doesn't affect just the individuals tested but those who hear their stories as well, including friends, family members, and acquaintances.

To understand this cycle, imagine that you have no symptoms and decide to undergo screening. Let's start with the most common test result: you are

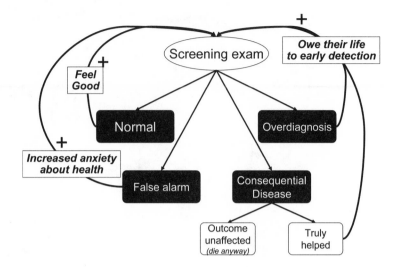

FIGURE 12.4 *The Self-reinforcing Cycle That Promotes*
*More Testing—Regardless of the Test Result*

found to be normal. To persuade you to be tested in the first place, someone (perhaps a doctor, a friend, the author of a magazine article, or the designer of an advertising campaign) suggested that something might be wrong with you, something that could eventually have grave consequences, despite your current lack of symptoms. But now that your results have come back normal and that possibility is off the table, you feel good. You, and others like you in similar situations, become enthusiastic about screening. It's easy to see how this works. Imagine hearing about a new brain cancer–screening campaign. There are campaigns like this. The Brain Tumor Foundation, for example, recently brought its mobile Road to Early Detection brain scanner to the U.S. Capitol, hoping to scan the brains of America's leaders looking for tumors (and, of course, to gather support for the program). Here's what it says on their Web site:

> It is a fact that over half of all brain tumor patients could have their tumors successfully removed for good if they are detected early, before physical symptoms become apparent. And, the only way to detect a tumor early is through the use of MRI brain scans. By providing the means to find and subsequently treat brain tumors early in their development, thousands of lives may be saved.
>
> We have grown accustomed to routinely checking for breast, colon, prostate and other cancers—why not brain tumors?[4]

How would you feel after reading something like that?

For one, you might start worrying that you have a brain tumor. You might worry even more if you heard of someone recently diagnosed with a brain tumor, perhaps a friend or perhaps a public figure (such as the late Senator Kennedy, who had been diagnosed a few months before the Road to Early Detection visited Washington). So you go for a scan and get a little nervous as your head goes inside. Your anxiety increases as you wait for the results. The possibility of a deadly cancer might seem more real. Now imagine you hear the result: you don't have brain cancer. You are relieved. You know you are healthy. Testing was a good thing because it reassured you of this fact. So it makes sense to do it again in the future to be sure you are still healthy. And it makes sense to recommend it to your friends.

But what has really happened? Basically, the system that promotes early diagnosis induced a measure of anxiety and then took it away. Some have pointed out that the reassurance is largely an illusion—a single normal screening exam has little effect on your overall chances of dying from cancer.[5] Nevertheless, any reassurance derived from the normal scan provides positive feedback for future testing. There is also a related phenomenon at work in this positive-feedback loop. Once your anxiety has been raised about a disease, you want to be sure you don't forgo the chance to avoid it in the future. In fact, if you don't get screened and you get sick, you think it will be your own fault.[6] This "anticipated regret" also promotes more testing.

Now consider a different test result: suppose you have a false alarm. False alarms, as you'll recall, are test results that are worrisome but that ultimately prove to be unfounded. These are false-positive results, and they are most common in cancer screening (making up somewhere around 5 to 15 percent of all results).[7] In this case, a false alarm would mean that your brain scan was abnormal in some way. There was a small mass that could be cancer. Pretty terrifying. For doctors to figure out exactly what the mass is, you have to have a biopsy. The surgeon has to drill a hole through your skull and use a very fine needle to take a piece of the mass. All goes well and the mass turns out not to be cancer after all. You feel an extraordinary sense of relief. You are immensely thankful to have dodged the bullet. (An oncologist friend of mine used to joke that we could make the entire population feel better if we told all of them that their tests showed they might have cancer and then a week or so later told them we'd been wrong.)

Interestingly, while you might think that a false alarm would discourage subsequent testing, few people are angered by the short-term anxiety. In a national survey that my coauthors and I conducted, more than 40 percent of Americans who had experienced a false alarm from a cancer screening test characterized the experience as "very scary" or "the scariest time of my life."

Yet looking back, almost every one said they were "glad" they had had the test.[8] The intense relief after a false alarm and the residual anxiety some people experience about their health[9] serve as positive feedback for more testing.

But what if it's not a false alarm? What if you learn you really have the disease; in this case, brain cancer? Even here you might be told there's some good news. The Web site for the Brain Tumor Foundation states that "it is a fact that over half of all brain tumor patients could have their brain tumors successfully removed for good if they are detected early." (Note: There is no reference for this claim, nor have I been able to find any data to support it—although it is perfectly plausible, if half of the patients were overdiagnosed.) So you go for surgery. If you do well, you assume that you owe your life to early detection. So does everyone else. That is the most powerful positive feedback for more testing. Of course, it is assumed that the tumor was destined to kill you. But the truth is that no one knows whether it was a deadly cancer or whether you were overdiagnosed.

And what is most ironic is that the more overdiagnosis a screening program causes, the more popular it becomes.[10] More overdiagnosis makes it increasingly likely that people will know others who have been diagnosed. This raises their personal sense of risk—so testing becomes all the more important. And an even more powerful reinforcement for screening is that more overdiagnosis also causes more people to believe they owe their lives, or the lives of those they know, to screening. Remember, overdiagnosed patients tend to do extraordinarily well, so it's easy to conclude that their lives were saved because their diseases were detected early. Once the cycle has begun, these influences will persist even if there are no other forces promoting screening (such as financial gain or true belief). This makes it difficult to back away from established tests, even when the medical community thinks it's the right thing to do. No matter what the experiences have been, the public tends to seek more testing.[11]

### *Hurricane prevention—an analogy for the dilemma of early diagnosis*

The idea that early diagnosis can do more harm than good is counterintuitive. Sometimes it helps to look elsewhere to get the big picture. A few years ago, following the terrible hurricane season of 2005, I read about an idea for preventing hurricanes. It struck me as a wonderful analogy for my profession's preferred approach to preventing disease. Here's an excerpt of the story that ran in the *Washington Post*:

> Moshe Alamaro has a modest proposal. Get a fleet of ocean barges and mount 10 or 20 jet engines—tails up—on each one. Fill the barges with

aviation fuel and tow them into the path of an oncoming hurricane. Light off the jets.

If everything goes as planned, the jets will trigger small tropical storms, "like backfires," Alamaro says, marginally lowering the surface ocean temperature and depriving the real hurricane of energy as it gets closer to shore.[12]

The engineers were proposing an idea analogous to one already in practice in the American West for fighting forest fires—a backfire. A backfire is a fire purposefully ignited in the wildfire's path. The rationale for a backfire is that it consumes the inputs a forest fire needs to continue to burn, namely, oxygen and fuel; the rationale for a "back-hurricane" is that it consumes the inputs a hurricane needs to continue to circulate (in this case, heat). Even a small disturbance might alter a hurricane's path.

It's an intriguing idea. The engineers acknowledged, however, that they were unsure if it would really work. Hurricanes are big by the time they hit the Gulf of Mexico—often hundreds of miles in diameter. They represent an overwhelming force. It would take a lot of back-hurricanes to do the job. The engineers recognized this. So they contemplated a different approach. Hurricanes are small when they form, usually off the coast of West Africa. Assuming they could get barges of jet fuel across the Atlantic in a timely manner, fewer back-hurricanes would be required to extinguish them there. In other words, they would be easier to deal with if they were caught early. Sound familiar? It's the fundamental rationale for early diagnosis.

To their credit, engineers recognized the side effect of this approach. Yes, they might be able to extinguish a catastrophic hurricane (such as Hurricane Katrina, which wiped out New Orleans, or the Great Hurricane of 1938, which wiped out much of New England), but they'd also extinguish the much more frequent hurricanes that were destined to simply dissipate over the North Atlantic.

"The trouble is that there's a trade-off between energy and information," [Kerry] Emanuel said. "The further in advance you do it, the smaller the energy you need but the more unpredictable the effect."

Unpredictable . . . as in they might alter the path of a hurricane destined for the North Atlantic and redirect it straight to Miami. That's the dilemma of early diagnosis.

# Pursuing Health with Less Diagnosis

I BELIEVE OVERDIAGNOSIS IS THE biggest problem posed by modern medicine. It is a problem relevant to virtually all medical conditions. It has led millions of people to become patients unnecessarily, to be made anxious about their health, to be treated needlessly, and to bear the inconvenience and financial burdens associated with overdiagnosis. It has added staggering costs to our already overburdened health-care system. And all of the forces that helped create and exacerbate the problem—financial gain, true belief, legal concerns, media messages, and self-reinforcing cycles—are powerful obstacles to fixing it.

It's tempting to conclude that the solution is simply to avoid doctors. But that would be the wrong conclusion. Let me remind you of what I said in the introduction. The question I'm raising is not whether you should seek out a doctor—and a diagnosis—when you are sick. Medical care offers ill patients a great deal. The question is about when you are well. How hard should doctors look for things to be wrong?

We must all view the dogma of early diagnosis more skeptically. I realize that may be a really tough paradigm shift. Just about everybody says that it is *always* in people's interest to detect health problems early. It just seems so obviously true. To suggest otherwise seems dangerous and irresponsible. But sometimes scientific paradigms simply need to change.

### Changing paradigms is challenging
To focus on writing this book, I took a sabbatical from my home institution and returned to the part of the country where I was raised, the Rocky Mountain West. One of the great things about getting away is meeting new people and learning new things. The combination can encourage you to think about things differently. I spent most of my sabbatical year at Montana State University in Bozeman, where I was exposed to a lot of geology. This is not surprising since the immediate area, the greater Yellowstone ecosystem, is filled with evidence of recent geologic activity, including volcanoes, earth-

quakes, and glaciers. But what was surprising is that something I learned there about the history of geology seemed to have parallels with the paradigm of early diagnosis.

If you have ever driven through eastern Washington State, you know that the landscape is pretty stark. It contains some of the most barren lands in our country; it's dry, rocky, and treeless. But it's decidedly not flat. Instead, it is laced with large braided channels, sometimes over a mile wide, that cut through solid rock. There are also immense potholes, narrow deep canyons, and remnants of huge waterfalls. What makes the area so unique is what you don't find: the substance needed to form these features, water.

J. Harlen Bretz was the first geologist to study this landscape. He called it "the channeled scablands," and he believed he knew what had created it: sudden massive flooding—flooding on a scale simply not seen anymore; flooding on a scale like that which would be created by dumping Lake Michigan on the state of Illinois over a matter of days. In 1923, Bretz published a paper outlining his argument. But the argument was heretical to the prevailing geologic paradigm. At the time, geologists believed that the world around them was the product of slow processes and weak forces that acted over long periods. Landscapes changed, but slowly, over hundreds of thousands of years. A theory that suggested a cataclysmic event, such as a flood of biblical proportions, was bound to provoke a hostile response from scientists whose life work was based on a fundamental belief in gradual change.

And it did. An emeritus professor of geology at the university in Montana described the reaction to Bretz's presentation at the 1927 meeting of the Geologic Society of America:

> A cabal of his more prominent detractors converted the occasion into what they called a debate, but it was more like an ambush. Some who were there described it as a lynching. Several of the prominent geologists in the audience denounced Bretz's ideas in terms so abrasive they were personal insults. It was, by all accounts, a shameful display, especially considering some of the most vocal detractors still had not visited the scablands and had no personal knowledge of those extraordinary landscapes. They based their arguments entirely on the received gospel of slow processes, weak forces, and plenty of time.[1]

As you may have surmised, the reason I tell this story is that Bretz's ideas were eventually shown to be correct. Joseph Pardee, a geologist working for the U.S. Geological Survey, discovered the source of the flood: Glacial Lake

Missoula, a huge lake in western Montana formed by ice dams during the ice age. The continental ice sheets had pushed south from Canada and blocked the headwaters of the Columbia River drainage. The water rose behind them, ultimately high enough (nearly two thousand feet deep) to float the dam away, releasing a massive flood. Amazingly, this cycle was repeated over and over, leading to roughly forty massive floods.

But it took decades for Bretz's idea to become widely accepted. Satellite imaging in the 1970s helped make the history of the floods more obvious. And once the idea was accepted, geologists found evidence of massive flooding resulting from failed ice dams in a number of other parts of the world.[2] Of course, Bretz's being right does not mean the geologic dogma is always wrong. Most geologic structures are the result of slow processes, weak forces, and plenty of time, but not always. Cataclysmic events do happen. So the truth is more nuanced.

I wanted to share Bretz's story to give you a sense of how difficult it is to change "scientific" paradigms. Just like geology, medicine has its own paradigms, and one of the most prominent is the belief in the value of early diagnosis. But a number of doctors have been raising questions about the paradigm of early diagnosis, some of them for decades. None is saying it's always wrong. There are definitely situations when it is better to treat a disease earlier rather than later. But the paradigm of early diagnosis is not always right, and it is less likely to be right as we look for earlier and earlier forms of disease.

In one respect, Bretz had it easy. The geologic paradigm of slow processes, weak forces, and plenty of time was confined to a small circle of scientists. In contrast, the paradigm of early diagnosis has been promulgated well beyond the medical community and is now widely accepted by the general public. So it is even more difficult to change. Recall what happened in 2009 when the U.S. Preventive Services Task Force suggested that women in their forties consider deferring mammography until age fifty and then undergoing screening every two years instead of every year. Within two weeks of that announcement, the Department of Health and Human Services disavowed the task force recommendations; task force members were hauled before Congress; and the Senate passed an amendment to require insurance coverage of mammography (as well as screening for lung and ovarian cancer—tests for which no credible evidence of benefit exists and which can cause substantial harm).[3]

### Needed: A healthy skepticism about early diagnosis

All of us need to view early diagnosis with a more critical eye and recognize that it can be a double-edged sword: it probably helps some, but it hurts others. My colleagues and I call this "healthy skepticism"—in this case, your skepticism can actually keep you healthy. To look at early diagnosis more critically, it helps to put it in perspective.

First, it is useful to start with some context—to understand why people get sick. The standard explanation invokes some combination of genetics and environment. Think of your genes as something you are not going to change (at least, it's not possible yet). Your environment (physical surroundings, what you eat, and so on) is more malleable. Some of it can't be changed, but much of it can be—particularly your personal habits, both good and bad. Of course, there's another reason why people get sick: bad luck. People with the same genetic makeup and living in the same environment may have different health outcomes. Chance certainly plays a role in who develops aggressive cancers, and the same is probably true for other diseases. Biologists might call this an unpredictable, idiosyncratic interaction of genetics and environment, but most of us would simply call it bad luck.

Understanding why people get sick is important so that everyone has realistic expectations of his or her own ability to affect future risk of disease. While some of it is within an individual's control, much of it is not. Even the disease that's considered the most avoidable—lung cancer—still occurs in people who have never smoked. It's also important so that everyone has realistic expectations of the ability of physicians to predict the future development of disease. Simply put, there are a lot of factors involved. This complexity limits the ultimate value of early diagnosis. The wild card of bad luck, in particular, makes it difficult to know who will benefit in the future from actions taken now.

Second, to place early diagnosis in its proper perspective, it is important to respect the role of symptoms. Early diagnosis occurs in both the presence and the absence of symptoms. But symptoms matter a lot. Because they give information about a person's present condition, they say something about the potential to benefit from intervention. The presence or absence of symptoms is a critical distinction in assessing the importance of an abnormality, because symptoms are one of the best predictors of serious problems.[4] This is not to say that all symptoms are harbingers of dire outcomes. But in general, a symptomatic individual with an abnormality is more likely to suffer an adverse outcome than an asymptomatic individual with the same abnormality. Furthermore, the presence of symptoms means there is room to get better. In a very real sense, patients with symptoms are experiencing adverse outcomes at that moment— and they are asking the doctors for help. This is in stark contrast to those who *might* experience adverse outcomes in the future but are currently well. The doctor offers help, but it is hard to make someone who is healthy feel better, and, unfortunately, it is easy to make them feel worse. Consequently, we need to think differently about these two groups of individuals.

The reason is simple: people with current symptoms can decide if an intervention is working. If your headache isn't better after you take medicine, you may decide the pills don't work. Alternatively, if you take the medicine and the headache goes away completely in twenty minutes, you may decide the drug is a winner. This kind of judgment is simply not possible with treatments that reduce the risk of future events. If you take a cholesterol medicine or are screened for cancer, for example, you won't feel your reduced risk of future heart attack or cancer death. That's why we need to be skeptical about broad claims about the value of early diagnosis. People experiencing symptoms can judge benefit on their own;[5] asymptomatic people cannot. And that's why I argue that careful evaluation, using randomized trials, is so important in determining the effectiveness of early diagnosis in asymptomatic persons.

### Recognize that while early may be good, earlier is not necessarily better

The early diagnosis paradigm is simple: the earlier that abnormalities are detected, the better. People tend to assume that the strategy to get the most benefit, then, is to catch abnormalities as early as possible. But as you now know, this is a recipe for overdiagnosis. The problem here is in the failure to distinguish between degrees of earliness. A more nuanced view is required: early may be good, but that doesn't mean earlier is better. In other words, there is almost certainly a point of negative returns, a degree of earliness that is too early because it labels too many people as sick and exposes too many low-risk people to the harms of treatment.

The obvious question is "Where is the point of negative returns?" Unfortunately, no one can answer that question precisely. But I can tell you the point at which we should start worrying about this question: when diagnoses are made in the absence of symptoms. Abnormalities or diseases diagnosed this early—that is, before symptoms occur—are not reliably destined *ever* to cause symptoms.

As a general rule, it's good to deal with symptomatic disease early.[6] Physicians would rather repair a deep laceration in the skin soon after it occurs than wait and treat infection when it sets in. We'd rather see patients earlier in the course of pneumonia than later when they develop difficulty breathing and low blood pressure. We'd rather see patients earlier in the course of their heart attacks than later when they develop dangerous heart rhythms and low blood pressure. And each of us would rather see a woman with a small breast lump than a woman who's waited and developed a large breast mass.

So when I suggest that we develop a healthy skepticism about early diagnosis, I am referring specifically to seeking diagnoses in the absence of symptoms, because that's when overdiagnosis can occur. I am not suggesting all diseases are curable after symptoms appear (most symptomatic lung and pancreatic cancers are not), nor am I suggesting that no diagnoses should be made in the absence of symptoms (severe high blood pressure should certainly be diagnosed). I'm simply suggesting that we should be most cautious about early diagnosis in those who feel well.

Many forces have combined to make medical care a more prominent part of all of our lives—even while we are well. Scientific advances mean more is possible; increased societal affluence means more is affordable. And the size of the market (that is, lots of healthy people) means there are strong economic incentives to promote early diagnostic services for the well. So it is important to think about how medical care might affect the experience of life. Do you see medical care as a way to deal with observable problems? Or as a vehicle to find and deal with problems you are not aware of? Of course, there are more than two choices—most of us want medical care to do both, to some extent. But there is a spectrum of strategies one might use to determine one's relationship to medical care. Each of us needs to consider where he wants to be on it.

Some may prefer to pursue health: to focus on feeling healthy and minimize medical contact while they are well. They may accept a slightly higher chance of death or disability to minimize the chance of medicalization, overdiagnosis, and overtreatment now. They prefer to reserve medical care for problems that are obvious to them.

Others may want to pursue disease: do everything they possibly can to be healthy in the future and to decrease their chances of experiencing death or disability—even with the knowledge that they are more likely to be diagnosed with disease, more likely to be frequently exposed to medical care, and more likely to suffer harm. They prefer to work to avoid death and choose to allow medical care to assume a larger role in their lives. Many view this as the best strategy to stay well. But it is difficult to promote wellness when actively looking for things to be wrong. In the effort to find out that everything is okay, people pursue early diagnosis. Ironically, this strategy increases the chances that they'll be told something is wrong.

In case it helps, here's how I think about it: To the extent that I have control over my cause of death, avoiding a heart-disease death, an aneurysm death, or a cancer death isn't my top priority. I'm more concerned about suffering a lingering cognitive decline in a long-term-care facility. And extending life is not the only outcome that matters to me. I place considerable value on feeling well: not being medicalized and not suffering the side effects of treatment any more than I need to.

Of course, different people will have different approaches to life. And individuals may feel differently about different diseases—particularly if some specific disease runs in the family.[7] Adding to that variability is the fact that people may feel differently at different points in life. When we have major responsibilities to others, such as young children, we are likely to place more value on the "staying alive" side of the equation. But later in life, we may place more value on "staying well." So we should expect that people will make different decisions about early diagnosis and that individuals' decisions may change over time. In short, there is no single right answer.

### *Seeing through persuasive messages*

If you decide that the best course of action is not always pursuing early diagnosis, then you will need to be prepared to do battle against the persistent messages in the culture persuading people of just the opposite. I know I touched on this earlier, but the issue is important enough—and the messages persuasive enough—that it's worth coming back to here. Many of these messages reflect belief, not data. Consider the following:

> *From your local television station:* It's easier and it's cheaper to stay healthy rather than get healthy, so use the 4NEWS Health Fair screening information to help stay at a good level of fitness. You're definitely going to be a lot better off—save a lot more money in the long run and keep on top of your health rather than trying to get better once you become sick.

> *From your local hospital:* Vascular disease can kill and cripple. DON'T BE A VICTIM. Are you at risk for stroke or aneurysm? Vascular screenings could save your life.

Assertions that early diagnosis saves lives or leads people to be better off should be viewed skeptically. They may be true, but they may not be. The only way to know is to have reliable data from a randomized trial.

Many messages overstate how common a disease is or how bad it is, including those messages put forth by disease advocacy groups:

*From a disease advocacy group:* Osteoporosis is a condition in which the bones become weak and can break from a minor fall or, in serious cases, from a simple action such as a sneeze. An estimated one in two women and one in four men over age fifty will have an osteoporosis-related fracture in their remaining lifetime. . . . If you have a family history of osteoporosis, you may be at risk. Make lifelong bone health a family tradition.

There are many ways to manipulate statistics to make diseases sound common or to make it sound like everyone is at risk when typically only a small group is affected. For example, the vast majority of osteoporosis fractures occur after age seventy-five or eighty. But statistics are often presented for people age fifty and over, making it sound like the big risk is coming soon, rather than twenty or thirty years in the future.

Still other messages highlight the tremendous improvements in survival:

*From a national news magazine:* If we find cancer early, 90 percent survive. If we find cancer late, 10 percent survive.

It is true that patients diagnosed early always have better survival statistics than those diagnosed late. And it's true that the survival statistics for many diseases have increased dramatically over the past fifty years. But none of this tells you that early diagnosis helps. Improved survival may simply reflect diagnosing people earlier in life; there's no delay in the time of their deaths, just a longer survival time from the point of diagnosis. Or it may represent an artifact of overdiagnosis; people who were never destined to die from the disease were diagnosed.

Other messages are emotionally compelling and use friends, family, acquaintances, or celebrities who "owe their lives" to early diagnosis:

*From a television news reporter and cancer survivor:* The first piece of advice I'd give to guys over forty-five is to get their prostate glands checked annually. That includes the PSA blood test and a digital rectal exam, where the doctor feels for lumps on the prostate. This is no time for modesty. Early detection can keep you from dying.

There are currently a lot of people who appear to be in this group. But that's the popularity paradox of screening: the more overdiagnosis that screening causes, the more people will feel they owe their lives to screening, and the more popular it will become. And you will never hear stories from people who were overdiagnosed, since it is impossible to know who they are.[8]

While the media is filled with persuasive messages about early diagnosis, the most persuasive ones may come from your doctor. Disagreeing with a doctor who is suggesting more diagnosis can be challenging. Some people may feel too intimidated to say no when offered a test. They may be afraid of making their doctors mad, of being called (or feeling) irresponsible, and they may worry that they will come to regret the decision in the future. The experience of one of my coauthors really highlights the challenges facing a patient who's trying to say no. And remember—she's a doctor.

This story is about my second pregnancy. But I have to start with my first: my daughter, Emma, was born six weeks early. She was bright yellow— caused by a high bilirubin related to bruising from her breech delivery— but otherwise perfect. She never needed oxygen support, was able to nurse on her second day, and her bilirubin started coming down in a few days. Looking back, I think Emma was ready to be born—this pregnancy just happened to be at the short end of the "normal" distribution of the length of pregnancies. But at the time it was pretty scary. Emma spent a week in the neonatal intensive care unit, and my heart stopped every time those alarm bells went off.

Two years later I was pregnant again. After initially being elated (and, of course, subsequently nauseated), I made my first prenatal visit to one of the "premier" obstetricians at our local medical center. She was worried. My first baby was premature; therefore I was at high risk. She wasn't buying any of this "short end of the normal distribution" stuff. She thought I should be seen in the high-risk clinic.

The more times she called me high risk, the more anxious I got. Despite my racing pulse and growing sweat stains, I remembered something. I am a researcher who studies risk. And I know that the first thing to do to understand a risk is to get some data. So, I asked some questions. "What do you mean 'high risk'? High risk for what?" The answer was "high risk of having a *seriously* premature baby." But when I asked for some numbers—specifically, the chances of having a seriously premature baby—she could not give me any. But she was certain it was very high.

And since I was high risk, I had to have high-risk treatment. So while it is not the usual practice to do a pelvic exam early in pregnancy, she suggested doing one. After completing the exam, she reported the cervix felt a little soft (of course, this is a very subjective finding—and since most women are never examined at this stage, I wonder if many obstetricians know exactly how a cervix *should* feel at this point). A soft cervix could mean trouble, so she then suggested a vaginal ultrasound to evaluate the length of the cervix—which was thought to be an excellent predictor of premature labor. I had the vaginal ultrasound (which demonstrated my cervical length was normal). However, the OB wanted to continue doing routine pelvic exams to pick up any sign of impending premature labor.

My husband, Steven (also a doctor and one of the other authors of this book), was helpful here—he convinced me to tell her to stop. He thought that it made no sense to do a test that couldn't be interpreted reliably, and he thought the exams were just making both of us really anxious.

So I told the doctor I didn't want any more of these routine exams. She agreed but made it clear that I should be prepared to accept the consequences (so now I would have to live with the fear of preterm labor *and* bearing the blame for not accepting monitoring if that happened). Of course, medicine currently has no effective therapy to prevent preterm labor, so it is hard to understand how this monitoring could help—and yet I now felt more vulnerable because I had refused recommended treatment.

Having refused to continue high-risk monitoring, I moved to the normal monitoring routine for pregnant women: weight and glucose testing. Again, my obstetrician was worried. Despite my terrible nausea and vomiting, I had gained a lot of weight. (Steven tried to be helpful in his annoying way—he told me not to worry, that the baby probably accounted for at least four pounds of my fifty-pound weight gain.)

Other than during pregnancy, I have never had a problem with weight, and I'd quickly lost the weight after Emma was born. But my OB warned me about the dangers of too much weight and went on to tell me how to avoid calories. I was starting to feel bad again. Then she told me I needed to do the glucose-tolerance test—although my sugar was currently normal. This would tell me whether I was at risk for diabetes during pregnancy.

Having read some of the guidelines about glucose testing and its unclear benefit, I asked if I really needed to have this done. She thought I was crazy: "You have gained so much weight, you are at high risk but refused monitoring exams, now you don't want the glucose-tolerance test—don't you care about your child?"

Ouch. That's a personal insult. Not that different from the reaction Bretz received in 1927. Lisa did the test. It was normal. So was her son, Eli, who was born at term. So everything turned out fine. But as she looks back on it, her pregnancy was a time of being seen as diseased and of being anxious—about both what could happen and being labeled a "difficult patient." Lisa's story highlights the resistance patients may face from their doctors if they choose not to undergo screening. It's easy for doctors to make their patients anxious about the dangers of refusing testing. But that doesn't mean the patients really are taking a dangerous course. While some doctors may discount the downsides of testing—including the time, the hassles, the emotional wear and tear, and the physical harms—these downsides are very real.

Not all doctors are like Lisa's. Many will be more open to a conservative approach to diagnosis than you might expect. Remember, our default assumption is that people want to be tested—that is, that they want to pursue disease. Those who prefer to pursue health should give their doctors permission not to search indiscriminately for things to be wrong. Such caution is relevant not only to screening, but also to efforts to establish exactly what is wrong when facing a minor problem (which is how we often stumble onto abnormalities, leading to more overdiagnosis). A patient who wants to pursue a more considered approach may not be seen by the doctor as confrontational but perhaps as a breath of fresh air. Both doctors and patients need to be educated that refusing testing is an acceptable approach.

### There's more to prevention than early diagnosis

One reason it is so hard to think more critically about early diagnosis is that it has become synonymous with preventive medicine. Preventive medicine is widely viewed as an unambiguous good—thus, early detection must be an unambiguous good. And it's hard to think critically about things that are assumed to be unambiguously good. So it's important to recognize that early detection is only one aspect of preventive medical care. In fact, some would argue that early diagnosis has nothing to do with prevention, since its whole purpose is to find disease, not prevent it. Of course, the idea is to find abnormalities early in their course and then prevent their consequences. But as you know, many of us harbor abnormalities that are not destined to produce consequences. So ironically, the fastest way to become sick is to become engaged in this type of preventive care.

Luckily, preventive medicine also involves health promotion. Think of health promotion as what your grandmother might have told you when you were young: don't smoke, eat your fruits and vegetables, and go play outside (with the hidden message: get some exercise and blow off some steam). Her idea was simple: lead a healthy life.

This is in stark contrast to early diagnosis. Early diagnosis is what a machine—usually interpreted by an overly cautious human—might tell you. Laboratory tests, X-rays and scans, and genetic tests are all about finding something wrong. But health promotion is more than an effort to extend life or to avoid disease and disability. That's because *health* means more than "absence of disease." Health is also about how people feel; it's a state of mind.

Thus health-promotion efforts need to be judged using a broader set of parameters than is traditionally used for medical care. My coauthors and I would rank highest those health-promotion efforts that lead people to feel more resilient, either physically or emotionally. By *resilient* I mean feeling strong, able to participate in and enjoy the life you lead—and capable of meeting and dealing with adversity when it comes.

Achieving this goal may require different behaviors in different people. And because *health* will invariably mean different things to different people, our ability to provide a scientific argument for specific strategies will always be somewhat limited. But I believe that, ironically, pursuing health requires not paying too much attention to it. Dwelling on the diseases we may develop in the future could become a real source of anxiety. It could lead us to seek too much medical care—which, of course, could lead to overdiagnosis.

And as you know, that's not the way to pursue health.

MY MOTHER DIED JUST AS I was completing this book, hence the dedication to her. But I should also acknowledge her contribution during life. While she was unable to provide any direct input (with the exception of some comic relief) to this book, she certainly laid the groundwork for my writing it. When I was a high school student, no one was harder on my writing than Mom. She made it clear that good writing didn't come easily but was the product of careful thought and constant revision. Perhaps more important, she was equally hard on the medical profession. When I was in college and, later, in medical school, she exposed me to the excesses in medicine she dealt with as member of the state's certificate-of-need program and as a hospital trustee during the 1970s ("Do we really need two CT scanners in this town?"). These influences ultimately set the stage for my writing this book.

While I take responsibility for all the words, I certainly can't take credit for all the ideas. This book would not have been possible without the work of others. I regret that their contribution is only acknowledged in the notes. A few have contributed to not only the underlying science but also the writing itself. My coauthors—Lisa Schwartz and Steve Woloshin—clearly fit in this category, as they have both performed considerable original research in the area and were involved in writing the entire book. I also want to acknowledge the more focused contributions of my colleagues Bill Black and Wylie Burke, whose research and feedback were invaluable to the sections dealing with radiology (chapters 3 and 7) and genetics (chapter 9).

Ideas and attention to the writing process are necessary ingredients for writing a book, but they are not sufficient. The final prerequisite is time: time to write, and time to think. I am indebted to the Department of Veterans Affairs—both its Health Services Research and Development Service and its local VA hospital in White River Junction—for supporting the sabbatical during which this book was written and, more broadly, for supporting my work over two decades. I particularly want to thank Gary DeGasta, our recently retired hospital director, who for twenty years acted on his vision of a small rural VA hospital, asking big questions about the U.S. health-care system.

Others also helped make my sabbatical happen. I appreciate the salary support provided by the Helmut Schumann Special Fellowship in Healthful Living, and the collegiality and office space provided by the Montana State University in Bozeman, Montana, and by the Gila Regional Medical Center in Silver City, New Mexico.

Finally, I am indebted to my wife, Linda, for both her tolerance (she has had to listen to some of these ideas ad nauseam) and her ability to give me space (sometimes when I'm writing, I'm not that "fun"). Her companionship provided me with the strength to persevere.

H. GILBERT WELCH
Thetford, Vermont

INTRODUCTION

1. Rob Stein, "Baby Boomers Appear to Be Less Healthy than Parents," *Washington Post,* April 20, 2007.


CHAPTER 1: GENESIS

1. It is true that even earlier, at the turn of the twentieth century, health officials began to seek out disease in healthy people who had had contact with tuberculosis patients. When effective treatments became available, these asymptomatic contacts may have been treated. And in the 1940s, the Pap smear was introduced as a way to diagnose and treat cervical cancer in asymptomatic individuals. In both cases, overdiagnosis undoubtedly occurred, but it was not the norm.

2. See F. H. Messerli, "This Day 50 Years Ago," *New England Journal of Medicine* 332 (1995): 1038–39.

3. See M. Moser, "Historical Perspectives on the Management of Hypertension," *Journal of Clinical Hypertension* 8 (2006):15–20, and R. C. Hamdy, "Hypertension: A Turning Point in the History of Medicine . . . and Mankind," *Southern Medical Journal* 94 (2001): 1045–47.

4. For example, see "Major Outcomes in High-Risk Hypertensive Patients Randomized to Angiotensin-converting Enzyme Inhibitor or Calcium Channel Blocker vs. Diuretic: The Antihypertensive and Lipid-Lowering Treatment to Prevent Heart Attack Trial (ALLHAT)," *Journal of the American Medical Association* 288 (2002): 2981–97, and N. S. Beckett, R. Peters, A. E. Fletcher, et al., "Treatment of Hypertension in Patients 80 Years of Age or Older," *New England Journal of Medicine* 358 (2008): 1887–98.

5. Iain Chalmers, "Joseph Asbury Bell and the Birth of Randomized Trials," www.james lindlibrary.org. Accessed May 16, 2008.

6. You might reasonably wonder why investigators need randomization to construct two groups of similar people; if a sixty-year-old male smoker with diabetes is enrolled in the Treatment group, then a sixty-year-old male smoker with diabetes should be enrolled in the No Treatment group. However, there are a number of problems with this approach. First, in terms of practicality, it is very difficult to accomplish. Second, it opens the door to either conscious or unconscious manipulation: investigators might skew the composition of the groups (e.g., putting the healthier people in the intervention group and the sicker people in the control group, which would make it appear that the intervention worked).

But the biggest problem is that investigators never fully know what factors need to be balanced in the two groups. While they can be certain that *some* factors will be important in determining health outcomes in a study (e.g., age, gender, smoking history, coexisting diseases), they can't be certain they know *all* the factors that will be important (e.g., the level of serum sodium, the genetic variant on the long arm of chromosome 11).

The beauty of randomization is that it is not only the best way to create groups that are similar in terms of known health factors but also the best way to create groups that are similar in terms of as-yet-unknown health factors.

7.  The data come from the Women's Health Initiative, a pair of large randomized trials run by the National Institutes of Health (NIH). Their Web site (http://www.nhlbi.nih .gov/whi/whi_faq.htm) summarizes the trials as follows: Compared with the placebo, estrogen plus progestin resulted in an increased risk of heart attack, stroke, blood clots and breast cancer, and a reduced risk of colon cancer and fractures. Compared with the placebo, estrogen alone resulted in an increased risk of stroke and blood clots, and a reduced risk of fractures. See "Risks and Benefits of Estrogen Plus Progestin in Healthy Postmenopausal Women," *Journal of the American Medical Association* 288 (2002): 321–33, and "Effects of Conjugated Equine Estrogen in Postmenopausal Women with Hysterectomy," *Journal of the American Medical Association* 291 (2004): 1701–12.

8.  There were seventy-three patients in the Treatment group and seventy patients in the group that received placebos. Note: The number of patients in the two groups was not exactly the same because individuals were assigned to either of the two groups by chance. Sometimes groups in randomized trials will be exactly the same size, but not often. If the assignment process is truly random, the chances are relatively low that the numbers will be exactly equal but quite high that they will be very similar in size.

9.  Veterans Administration Cooperative Study Group on Antihypertensive Agents, "Effects of Treatment on Morbidity in Hypertension," *Journal of the American Medical Association* 202 (1967): 1028–34. Readers can easily calculate the total number of patients experiencing events in the tally sheet by looking at table 4 in the article. However, it would take considerable effort to re-create the categorization of events shown here. Clinicians looking at the original article should know that I did my best to construct clinically meaningful categories for readers based on the individual listing of all twenty-nine patient events in tables 5 and 6. Full disclosure: I also included the one transient ischemic attack as a stroke, and the one cotton-wool exudate as a retinal hemorrhage. More than you wanted to know.

10.  "Effects of Treatment on Morbidity in Hypertension: II. Results in Patients with Diastolic Blood Pressure Averaging 90 through 114 mm Hg," *Journal of the American Medical Association* 213 (1970): 1143–52.

11.  J. D. Neaton, R. H. Grimm Jr., R. J. Prineas, et al., "Treatment of Mild Hypertension Study: Final Results," *Journal of the American Medical Association* 270 (1993): 713–24.

12.  Lest you think I made a mistake, here's the place rounding rears its ugly head. The actual chance of benefit is 5.6 percent, not 6 percent. Thus the number needed to treat is closer to 18.

13.  SHEP Cooperative Research Group, "Prevention of Stroke by Antihypertensive Drug Treatment in Older Persons with Isolated Systolic Hypertension: Final Results of the Systolic Hypertension in the Elderly Program (SHEP)," *Journal of the American Medical Association* 265 (1991): 3255–64.

14.  E. Arias, "United States Life Tables, 2003," *National Vital Statistics Reports* 54. Hyattsville, MD: National Center for Health Statistics, 2006.

15.  Many legitimate questions are raised by Mr. Bailey's story. First, how well did he understand the benefit of treatment? Second, did I adequately communicate that there

were other treatment options? For example, instead of forgoing treatment altogether, we could have tried a different drug, or the same drug at a lower dose, or the same drug but only while the weather was cool. Finally, might new information have changed his decision? Since then there has been another randomized trial of the treatment of hypertension in the elderly; for example, see Beckett et al., "Treatment of Hypertension." Unfortunately, that study combined elderly patients with mild diastolic hypertension with others who had isolated systolic hypertension (people like Mr. Bailey). Among all patients, it found about a 5 percent chance of benefit, but here the benefit was avoiding death (for any reason). Knowing these data might have changed Mr. Bailey's decision. It also might have affected me, since the study measured all of the patients' systolic pressure while they were standing and did not treat patients whose standing systolic pressure was below 140, in an effort to avoid the kind of episode that happened to Mr. Bailey.

16. It's likely that raising blood pressure targets (the numbers we shoot for with therapy) would reduce the problems of light-headedness, fainting, and falls. The target pressure for the above study was 150/80.

## CHAPTER 2: WE CHANGE THE RULES

1. "Report of the Expert Committee on the Diagnosis and Classification of Diabetes Mellitus," *Diabetes Care* 20 (1997): 1183.

2. L. M. Schwartz and S. Woloshin, "Changing Disease Definitions: Implications on Disease Prevalence," *Effective Clinical Practice* 2 (1999): 76–85.

3. Action to Control Cardiovascular Risk in Diabetes Study Group, "Effects of Intensive Glucose Lowering in Type 2 Diabetes," *New England Journal of Medicine* 358 (2008): 2545–59.

4. I wish there weren't more complexity, but there is. Although the diagnosis of diabetes is made using fasting glucose levels, therapy is typically directed toward average glucose levels. The way we measure average glucose levels is by measuring the amount of glycosylated hemoglobin, better known as hemoglobin A1c. The goal for the intensive-therapy group was a hemoglobin A1c of less than 6. Half of the patients made it to less than 6.4. This corresponds to an average blood sugar of 140 (or 127 or 132 or 150, depending on which Web calculator you use). I believe (and hope) that the distinction between how we diagnose the disease and how we guide therapy will ultimately disappear, and we will diagnose and treat diabetes based on hemoglobin A1c.

5. The press release can be accessed at http://www.nih.gov/news/health/feb2008/nhlbi-06 .htm.

6. For more on the change threshold, compare "The Fifth Report of the Joint National Committee on Detection, Evaluation, and Treatment of High Blood Pressure" in *Archives of Internal Medicine* 153 (1993): 154–83 with "The Sixth Report of the Joint National Committee on Prevention, Detection, Evaluation, and Treatment of High Blood Pressure" in *Archives of Internal Medicine* 157 (1997): 2413–46.

7. Schwartz and Woloshin, "Changing Disease Definitions."

8. J. Downs, M. Clearfield, S. Weis, et al., "Primary Prevention of Acute Coronary Events with Lovastatin in Men and Women with Average Cholesterol Levels: Results of AFCAPS/TexCAPS," *Journal of the American Medical Association* 179 (1998): 1615–22.

9.   Note that this evidence is much weaker than the evidence for secondary prevention—that is, the proven benefits of lowering cholesterol in those who have already had heart attacks (a reduction of heart-attack deaths). This study showed no difference in death from heart attacks (only a difference in the combined events).

10.  Schwartz and Woloshin, "Changing Disease Definitions."

11.  Healthy bones block X-rays. So the bones you see on an X-ray actually demonstrate the radiation that was blocked by the bones and didn't get to the film. Bone mineral density testing measures the extent to which the X-rays are blocked by a bone. The more the X-rays are blocked, the denser the bone must be.

12.  This might be the T score for a large-boned, physically active woman in her twenties. Could be my daughter's T score—were she willing to pay for the test.

13.  M. B. Herndon, L. M. Schwartz, S. Woloshin, et al., "Implications of Expanding Disease Definitions: The Case of Osteoporosis," *Health Affairs* 26 (2007): 1702–11.

14.  Search for James R. Gavin, chair of Expert Committee on the Diagnosis and Classification of Diabetes Mellitus, on http://www.cspinet.org/cgi-bin/integrity.cgi.

15.  Duff Wilson, "New Blood-pressure Guidelines Pay Off—for Drug Companies," *Seattle Times,* June 26, 2005; see http://seattletimes.nwsource.com/html/health/sick1.html.

16.  D. Ricks and R. Rabin, "Cholesterol Guidelines: Drug Panelists' Links under Fire," *Newsday*, July 15, 2004.

17.  Susan Kelleher, "Disease Expands Through Marriage of Marketing and Machines," *Seattle Times,* June 26, 2005; see http://seattletimes.nwsource.com/html/health/sick3.html.

18.  S. R. Cummings, D. M. Black, D. E. Thompson, et al., "Effect of Alendronate on Risk of Fracture in Women with Low Bone Density But Without Vertebral Fractures: Results from the Fracture Intervention Trial," *Journal of the American Medical Association* 280 (1998): 2077–82.

19.  M. Etminan, K. Aminzadeh, I. R. Matthew, and J. M. Brophy, "Use of Oral Bisphosphonates and the Risk of Aseptic Osteonecrosis: A Nested Case-control Study," *Journal of Rheumatology* 35 (2008): 691–95.

20.  Trial of Preventing Hypertension (TROPHY) Study Investigators, "Feasibility of treating Prehypertension with an Angiotensin-receptor Blocker," *New England Journal of Medicine* 354 (2006): 1685–97.

21.  Schwartz and Woloshin, "Changing Disease Definitions."

22.  See http://www.diabetes.org/pre-diabetes.jsp.

23.  For the media's reporting of this, see http://www.msnbc.msn.com/id/25556140/. For the academy's report, see S. R. Daniels, F. R. Greer, and the Committee on Nutrition, "Lipid Screening and Cardiovascular Health in Childhood," *Pediatrics* 122 (2008): 198–208; http://www.pediatrics.org/cgi/content/full/122/1/198.

24.  An alternative treatment threshold also qualifies: a ten-year probability of a major osteoporosis-related fracture of greater than 20 percent. For the entire guideline see the National Osteoporosis Foundation's "Clinician's Guide to Prevention and Treatment of osteoporosis," 2008, National Osteoporosis Foundation, Washington, DC; Web site http://www.nof.org/professionals/NOF_Clinicians_Guide.pdf.

25.  You can view the calculator yourself at http://www.shef.ac.uk/FRAX/tool.jsp?location Value=9.

CHAPTER 3: WE ARE ABLE TO SEE MORE

1.  J. M. Gwaltney, C. D. Phillips, R. D. Miller, and D. K. Riker, "Computer Tomographic Study of the Common Cold," *New England Journal of Medicine* 330 (1994): 25–30.

2.  IMV Medical Information Division, http://www.marketresearch.com/vendors/view vendor.asp?SID=22207180-472843397.

3.  David J. Brenner and Eric J. Hall, "Computed Tomography—an Increasing Source of Radiation Exposure," *New England Journal of Medicine* 357 (2007): 2277–84.

4.  These data come from our shop—the Dartmouth Institute for Health Policy and Clinical Practice—which has been collecting and analyzing Medicare data since the mid-1980s. These are Part B data for 1991 and 2006. For those looking for a denominator for these counts, it has actually shrunk a tiny bit as more beneficiaries left Part B for HMOs over the period (27,300,000 in 1991 and 26,300,000 in 2006).

5.  K. D. Hopper, J. R. Landis, J. W. Meilstrup, et al., "The Prevalence of Asymptomatic Gallstones in the General Population," *Investigative Radiology* 26 (1991): 939–45.

6.  The data presented here are from J. Kornick, E. Trefelner, S. McCarthy, et al., "Meniscal Abnormalities in the Asymptomatic Population at MR Imaging," *Radiology* 177 (1990): 463–65. The study was repeated some eighteen years later and found essentially the same thing (although the authors of the second study inexplicably failed to acknowledge the work of the first). See M. Englund, A. Guermazi, D. Gale, et al., "Incidental Meniscal Findings on Knee MRI in Middle-aged and Elderly Persons," *New England Journal of Medicine* 359 (2008): 1108–15. The second study took a random sample of the people in the Framingham Heart Study and looked at somewhat more severe injuries: either meniscal tears or meniscal destruction. Here is the approximate prevalence of both by age and gender:

|  | **Proportion with Meniscal Tear or Destruction** | |
| --- | :---: | :---: |
| **Age Group** | **Men** | **Women** |
| 50–59 years | 32% | 19% |
| 60–69 years | 46% | 40% |
| 70–90 years | 56% | 51% |

7.  M. C. Jensen, M. N. Brant-Zawadski, N. Obuchowski, et al., "Magnetic Resonance Imaging of the Lumbar Spine in People Without Back Pain," *New England Journal of Medicine* 331 (1994): 69–73.

8.  A. Kirkley, T. B. Birmingham, R. B. Litchfield, et al., "A Randomized Trial of Arthroscopic Surgery for Osteoarthritis of the Knee," *New England Journal of Medicine* 359 (2008): 1097–1107.

9.  R. G. Marx, "Arthroscopic Surgery for Osteoarthritis of the Knee?" *New England Journal of Medicine* 359 (2008): 1169–70.

10. The Framingham Heart Study was initiated in 1948 and was the first trial to document the basic risk factors for heart attacks: smoking, high blood pressure, high cholesterol, and so on. The participants in the stroke study were actually the offspring of the original participants. The prevalence of stroke by age group shown in the graph reflects the com-

bined findings in men and women (the differences by gender were small and inconsistent—in some age groups, the stroke prevalence was slightly higher in men, in others it was slightly higher in women). See R. R. Das, S. Seshadri, A. S. Beiser, et al., "Prevalence and Correlates of Silent Cerebral Infarcts in the Framingham Offspring Study," *Stroke* 39 (2008): 2929–35.

11.  R. Davis, "The Inside Story," *USA Today*, August 25, 2000.

12.  C. D. Furtado, D. A. Aguirre, C. B. Sirlin, et al., "Whole-body CT Screening: Spectrum of Findings and Recommendations in 1192 Patients," *Radiology* 237 (2005): 385–94.

13.  B. Mandelbrot, *The Fractal Geometry of Nature,* revised edition (New York: W. H. Freeman and Company, 1983), 116.

14.  And in Utah (as well as in other states in the intermountain west) you will also have to struggle with the question of when to make this determination. In May, some lakes will still be under snow; by September, some will have dried up. By the way, this exercise need not be limited to islands or lakes. The same issues come up when counting rivers or mountain peaks . . .

15.  F. A. Lederle, J. M. Walker, and D. B. Reinke, "Selective Screening for Abdominal Aortic Aneurysms with Physical Examination and Ultrasound," *Archives of Internal Medicine* 148 (1988): 1753–56.

16.  L. J. Melton, L. K. Bickerstaff, L. H. Hollier, et al., "Changing Incidence of Abdominal Aortic Aneurysms: A Population-based Study," *American Journal of Epidemiology* 120 (1984): 379–86.

17.  R. F. Gillum, "Epidemiology of Aortic Aneurysm in the United States," *Journal of Clinical Epidemiology* 48 (1995): 1289–98.

18.  W. H. Geerts, K. I. Code, R. M. Jay, et al., "A Prospective Study of Venous Thromboembolism after Major Trauma," *New England Journal of Medicine* 331 (1994): 1601–06.

19.  K. M. Moser, P. F. Fedullo, J. K. LitteJohn, et al., "Frequent Asymptomatic Pulmonary Embolism in Patients with Deep Venous Thrombosis," *Journal of the American Medical Association* 271 (1994): 223–25.

20.  D. R. Anderson, S. R. Kahn, M. A. Rodger, et al., "Computed Tomographic Pulmonary Angiography vs. Ventilation-perfusion Lung Scanning in Patients with Suspected Pulmonary Embolism: A Randomized Controlled Trial," *Journal of the American Medical Association* 298 (2007): 2743–53.

21.  N. A. DeMonaco, Q. Dang, W. N. Kapoor, et al., "Pulmonary Embolism Incidence Is Increasing with Use of Spiral Computed Tomography," *American Journal of Medicine* 12 (2008): 611–17.

22.  One physician reading this thought the word *illogical* was a little strong. He pointed out that it is not totally illogical to look for a major abnormality even in a setting where it's very unlikely. Of course, whether it is illogical or not hinges on just how unlikely the abnormality might be. This is a perfect example of why medicine is (and always will be) full of judgment calls. We both agree, however, that the problem of overdiagnosis arises when we look for a major abnormality and find something mildly abnormal (an ambiguous finding) or something totally unexpected (a surprise finding).

23.  I actually described this process in an introduction to an editorial on informed choice; see H. G. Welch, "Informed Choice in Cancer Screening," *Journal of the American Medical Association* 285 (2001): 2776–78.

CHAPTER 4: WE LOOK HARDER FOR PROSTATE CANCER

1. All the data in this and the subsequent paragraph can be found at http://seer.cancer.gov/, the federal government's program to track national cancer statistics.

2. J. E. Montie, D. P. Wood, J. E. Pontes, et al., "Adenocarcinoma of the Prostate in Cysto-prostatectomy Specimens Removed for Bladder Cancer," *Cancer* 63 (1989): 381–85. In this study, the pathologists examined the prostate every five millimeters, or about ten tissue slices per prostate (the typical prostate is about fifty millimeters long). If they had taken slices every two millimeters (that is, examined twenty-five slices), they might have found more cancer.

3. W. A. Sakr, D. J. Grignon, G. P. Haas, et al., "Age and Racial Distribution of Prostatic Intraepithelial Neoplasia," *European Urology* 30 (1996): 138–44. In this study, the pathologists also examined ten to fourteen slices per prostate. Reflecting the racial mix of Wayne County, about 60 percent of these men were black (who are more likely than whites to die from prostate cancer). However, the white/black differences they reported were small (≤ 6 percentage points within each age category). So the data reported here combine both groups.

4. It's tempting to think that the difference between the reservoir of prevalent prostate cancer in older men (to use round numbers, let's say 50 percent) and their lifetime risk of prostate cancer death (3 percent) would *exactly* reflect the potential proportion of older men who could be overdiagnosed ( 50 percent – 3 percent = 47 percent at risk of being overdiagnosed). But the comparison of the disease reservoir with the lifetime risk of death gives you a sense of the potential magnitude of overdiagnosis, not a precise estimate.

5. There is a broad range of prostate size. This calculation is based on a gland five centimeters in diameter.

6. In each of the three studies, the researchers took the higher number of biopsies (eleven, twelve, or thirteen, depending on the study). They then compared the proportion of men who were found to have prostate cancer using the standard six needle biopsies (the sextant biopsy) with the proportion of men who were found to have prostate cancer using the larger number of biopsies. For the value added of eleven vs. six biopsies, see R. J. Babaian, A. Toi, K. Kamoi, et al., "A Comparative Analysis of Sextant and an Extended 11-core Multisite Directed Biopsy Strategy," *Journal of Urology* 163 (2000): 152–57. For twelve vs. six, see G. C. Durkan, N. Sheikh, P. Johnson, et al., "Improving Prostate Cancer Detection with an Extended-core Transrectal Ultrasonography-guided Prostate Biopsy Protocol," *British Journal of Urology International* 89 (2002): 33–39. For thirteen vs. six, see L. A. Eskew, R. L. Bare, and D. L. McCullough, "Systematic 5 Region Prostate Biopsy Is Superior to Sextant Method for Diagnosing Carcinoma of the Prostate," *Journal of Urology* 157 (1997): 199–202.

7. See N. Fleshner and L. Klotz, "Role of 'Saturation Biopsy' in the Detection of Prostate Cancer among Difficult Diagnostic Cases," *Urology* 60 (2002): 93–97.

8. These yields come from two publications reporting on the same study. The yield for PSAs > 4 come from the placebo group in the trial of finasteride to reduce prostate cancer (see table 1, biopsy performed for cause, in I. M. Thompson, P. J. Goodman, C. M. Tangen, et al., "The Influence of Finasteride on the Development of Prostate Cancer," *New England Journal of Medicine* 349 (2003): 215–24). The yield for PSA ≤ 4 also come from the placebo group in the same trial but is reported in a separate publication (see I. M. Thompson, D. K. Pauler, P. J. Goodman, et al., "Prevalence of Prostate Cancer among

Men with a Prostate-Specific Antigen Level <=4.0 ng per Milliliter," *New England Journal of Medicine* 350 (2004): 2239–46).

9.  The data on the distribution of PSA in the general population come from work by my coauthors and me; see H. G. Welch, L. M. Schwartz, and S. Woloshin, "Prostate-specific Antigen Levels in the United States: Implications of Various Definitions for Abnormal," *Journal of the National Cancer Institute* 97 (2005): 1132–37.

10. The graph shows the estimated number of sixty- to sixty-nine-year-old males in the United States who would be diagnosed with prostate cancer if all were screened at a single point in time but using different rules to define abnormal PSA. For context, there are about eleven million men in this age group. The estimates are based on two inputs: (1) how many have abnormal PSAs under the various definitions of abnormal (from reference 9) and (2) how often prostate cancer is detected at various PSA levels (from reference 8).

11. W. J. Mooi and D. S. Peeper, "Oncogene-induced Cell Senescence—Halting on the Road to Cancer," *New England Journal of Medicine* 355 (2006): 1037–46; J. Folkman and R. Kalluri, "Cancer Without Disease," *Nature* 427 (2004): 787; M. Serrano, "Cancer Regression by Senescence," *New England Journal of Medicine* 356 (2007): 1996–97.

12. This is the pattern one of my colleagues and I reported for a rare form of esophageal cancer. See H. Pohl and H. G. Welch, "The Role of Overdiagnosis and Reclassification in the Marked Increase of Esophageal Adenocarcinoma Incidence," *Journal of the National Cancer Institute* 97 (2005): 142–46.

13. SEER is the federal government's primary effort to collect and report on cancer incidence, initial treatment, and survival. This database includes information from cancer registries in the states of Connecticut, Iowa, New Mexico, Utah, Hawaii, and the metropolitan areas of Detroit, San Francisco, Seattle–Puget Sound, and Atlanta. Together these areas represent approximately 10 percent of the U.S. population.

14. R. M. Merrill, E. J. Feuer, J. L. Warren, et al., "Role of Transurethral Resection of the Prostate in Population-based Prostate Cancer Incidence Rates," *American Journal of Epidemiology* 150 (1999): 848–60.

15. H. G. Welch and P. C. Albertsen, "Prostate Cancer Diagnosis and Treatment After the Introduction of Prostate-Specific Antigen Screening: 1986–2005," *Journal of the National Cancer Institute,* August 31, 2009 (Epub).

16. These data come from a variety of sources. Data on inpatient mortality following prostatectomy come from http://hcupnet.ahrq.gov/ (last accessed September 21, 2008); note that thirty-day mortality will be higher. Quality-of-life data come from A. L. Potosky, J. Legler, P. C. Albertsen, et al., "Health Outcomes after Prostatectomy or Radiotherapy for Prostate Cancer: Results from the Prostate Cancer Outcomes Study," *Journal of the National Cancer Institute* 92 (2000): 1582–92; and M. G. Sanda, R. L. Dunn, J. Michalski, et al., "Quality of Life and Satisfaction with Outcome among Prostate Cancer Survivors," *New England Journal of Medicine* 358 (2008): 1250–61.

17. These recommendations (see http://www.ahrq.gov/clinic/uspstf/uspsprca.htm; last accessed 10/3/08) were made before the 2009 publication of the two randomized trials discussed in the next section. But I doubt the trial results will change the recommendations much—screening will still be considered a difficult call (at best) for middle-aged men and a very unfavorable trade-off for elderly men.

18. These recommendations were made after the publication of the two randomized trials;

see http://www.cancer.org/docroot/CRI/content/CRI_2_6x_Prostate_Cancer_Early _Detection .asp?sitearea=&level= (last accessed 4/12/10).

19. G. L. Andriole, R. L. Grubb, S. S. Buys, et al., for the PLCO Project Team, "Mortality Results from a Randomized Prostate-Cancer Screening Trial," *New England Journal of Medicine* 360 (2009): 1310–19.

20. F. H. Schroder, J. Hugosson, M. J. Roobol, et al., for the ERSPC Investigators, "Screening and Prostate-Cancer Mortality in a Randomized European Study," *New England Journal of Medicine* 360 (2009): 1320–28.

21. To understand why screening might increase prostate cancer mortality, you need to know how prostate cancers deaths are counted in a randomized trial of screening. Prostate cancer deaths include not only the number of deaths from metastatic prostate cancer (which screening could not plausibly increase) but also the number of deaths from the treatment of prostate cancer (which, because it leads more men to be diagnosed, screening could easily increase).

22. As a starting point, I assume there are deaths averted—that is, I start with the European study, not the U.S. study. These data show one death averted to forty-eight additional diagnoses (which I rounded to one to fifty). Some would correctly point out that there is a reason to believe that fifty is an overestimate. Additional diagnoses may not all represent overdiagnosis—the passage of time may demonstrate the appearance of "catch-up" cancers in the control group. However, a prior publication by the European group did estimate the proportion of patients overdiagnosed in the screened group at 48 percent (see G. Draisma, R. Boer, S. J. Otto, et al., "Lead Times and Overdetection due to Prostate-specific Antigen Screening," *Journal of the National Cancer Institute* 95 (2003): 868–78). Applying this estimate to the 82/1,000 overall incidence in the screened group would suggest an overdiagnosis rate of 39/1,000, or 55 overdiagnosed men per one death averted (equals the product of the number needed to screen to prevent one prostate cancer death and the overdiagnosis rate: = 1410 × 39/1000).

Others would correctly point out that there are two reasons to believe that fifty is an underestimate of overdiagnosis in the United States. First, the European study represents less intense screening than is done in this county: the European study screened every four years, the U.S. practice is to screen annually, which can only increase the amount of overdiagnosis. Second, there is uncertainty about the death benefit: obviously, the less benefit, the lower the death-averted-to-overdiagnosis ratio (at zero benefit, it is one to infinity). To accommodate both concerns, my suggestion is to consider a range: for every man who benefits by avoiding a prostate cancer death, somewhere between thirty and a hundred are harmed by overdiagnosis and treated needlessly.

23. A. Bill-Axelson, L. Holmberg, F. Filén, et al., for the Scandinavian Prostate Cancer Group Study Number 4, "Radical Prostatectomy Versus Watchful Waiting in Localized Prostate Cancer: The Scandinavian Prostate Cancer Group-4 Randomized Trial," *Journal of the National Cancer Institute* 100 (2008): 1144–54; A. V. D'Amico, M. H. Chen, A. A. Renshaw, et al., "Androgen Suppression and Radiation vs. Radiation Alone for Prostate Cancer: A Randomized Trial," *Journal of the American Medical Association* 299 (2008): 289–95; B. Schmitt, C. Bennett, J. Seidenfeld, et al., "Maximal Androgen Blockade for Advanced Prostate Cancer," *Cochrane Database of Systematic Reviews* 2000, issue 2; DOI: 10.1002/14651858.CD001526.

24. Richard J. Ablin, "The Great Prostate Mistake," *New York Times,* March 10, 2010; http://www.nytimes.com/2010/03/10/opinion/10Ablin.html?pa.

CHAPTER 5: WE LOOK HARDER FOR OTHER CANCERS

1.  The thyroid is a gland in the lower neck; it makes thyroid hormone, which regulates a number of metabolic processes.

2.  S. Ezzat, D. A. Sarti, D. R. Cain, et al., "Thyroid Incidentalomas: Prevalence by Palpation and Ultrasonography," *Archives of Internal Medicine* 154 (1994): 1838–40.

3.  The autopsies were consecutive, which means every time there was an autopsy in the hospital the researchers did a systematic exam of the thyroid. This implies that the subjects were not selected for some unusual quality. See H. R. Harach, K. O. Franssila, and V. Wasenius, "Occult Papillary Carcinoma of the Thyroid: A 'Normal' Finding in Finland. A Systematic Autopsy Study," *Cancer* 56 (1985): 531–38.

4.  Their reasoning went something like this: They figured that since the slices were being made every two millimeters, any cancer larger than that could not be missed. But how about a one-millimeter cancer? Sometimes they would catch it in the slice, sometimes it would be in between. If the slices were every two millimeters, then roughly half the time they would cut through a one-millimeter cancer. A more formal explanation: the probability of detecting a small cancer is equal to its diameter divided by the distance between slices (in this case 1mm/2mm = 0.5). In other words, they were only finding half of the one-millimeter cancers. They were finding much smaller cancers as well, some as small as two-tenths of a millimeter. How many of these were they missing? Using the same reasoning, they were finding 10 percent (0.2mm/2mm = 0.1) and were missing 90 percent. For a more complete discussion of their reasoning (as well as some diagrams to illustrate what is going on), see H. G. Welch, *Should I Be Tested for Cancer?* (Berkeley: University of California Press, 2004), 79–82.

5.  See the *Guide to Clinical Preventive Services,* second edition, 1996, http://www.ahrq.gov/clinic/2ndcps/thyrdcan.pdf.

6.  This increase is observed in the Part B claims of Medicare for neck ultrasounds (CPT 76536). (This is data we have maintained at Dartmouth since 1991.)

7.  L. Davies and H. G. Welch, "The Increasing Incidence of Thyroid Cancer in the United States, 1973–2002," *Journal of the American Medical Association* 295 (2006): 2164–67.

8.  H. G. Welch, S. Woloshin, and L. M. Schwartz, "Skin Biopsy Rates and Incidence of Melanoma: Population Based Ecological Study," *British Medical Journal* 331 (2005): 481–84.

9.  See R. A. Swerlick and S. Chen, "The Melanoma Epidemic: More Apparent than Real?" *Mayo Clinic Proceedings* 72 (1997): 559–64; A. Florez and M. Cruces, "Melanoma Epidemic: True or False?" *International Journal of Dermatology* 43 (2004): 405–7; F. C. Beddingfield, "The Melanoma Epidemic: Res Ipsa Loquitur," *Oncologist* 8 (2003): 459–65.

10. See W. C. Black, "Lung Cancer," in B. S. Kramer, J. K. Gohagan, and P. C. Prorok, eds., *Cancer Screening: Theory and Practice* (New York: Marcel Dekker, 1999).

11. P. Marcus, E. Bergstralh, M. Zweig, et al., "Extended Lung Cancer Incidence Follow-up in the Mayo Lung Project and Overdiagnosis," *Journal of the National Cancer Institute* 98 (2006): 748–56.

12. R. Doll and A. B. Hill, "Lung Cancer and Other Causes of Death in Relation to Smoking; a Second Report on the Mortality of British Doctors," *British Medical Journal* 2 (1956): 1071–81.

13. S. Sone, F. Li, Z. Yang, et al., "Results of Three-year Mass Screening Programme for Lung Cancer Using Mobile Low-dose Spiral Computed Tomography Scanner," *British Journal of Cancer* 84 (2001): 25–32.

14. I pieced this story together from news reports at the time. See Irwin Block, "Mulroney

Surgery 'Successful,'" *Montreal Gazette,* March 16, 2005; and Philip Authier, "Mulroney Sent Home to Recover," *Montreal Gazette,* June 25, 2005. I attempted to confirm the details (and learn whether he had wanted to be screened or whether his doctors had recommended it) from his staff, but they chose not to respond.

15. For historical trends see http://seer.cancer.gov/csr/1973_1998/, Table I-3: Summary of Changes in Cancer Incidence and Mortality 1950–1998. SEER doesn't report these anymore (I don't know why), but as you can see in the graph, both cervical cancer incidence and mortality have only declined further since 1998.

16. A. M. Kavanagh, G. Santow, and H. Mitchell, "Consequences of Current Patterns of Pap Smear and Colposcopy Use," *Journal of Medical Screening* 3 (1996): 29–34.

17. See http://www.acog.org/departments/dept_notice.cfm?recno=20&bulletin=5021.

18. W. F. Whitmore Jr., "Consensus Development Conference on the Management of Clinically Localized Prostate Cancer. Overview: Historical and Contemporary," *National Cancer Institute Monographs* 7 (1988): 7–11.

## CHAPTER 6: WE LOOK HARDER FOR BREAST CANCER

1. See "The Politics of Mammography Screening: A History" in *Healthfacts,* June 1992; http://findarticles.com/p/articles/mi_m0815/is_n157_v17/ai_13217094/.

2. See A. B. Miller, C. J. Baines, T. To, et al., "Canadian National Breast Screening Study: 1. Breast Cancer Detection and Death Rates among Women Aged 40 to 49 Years," *Canadian Medical Association Journal* 147 (1992): 1459–76.

3. See S. W. Fletcher, W. Black, R. Harris, et al., "Report of the International Workshop on Screening for Breast Cancer," *Journal of the National Cancer Institute* 85 (1993): 1644–56.

4. Although I remember much of the story as it unfolded, I am indebted to Suzanne Fletcher for putting it down on paper. See S. W. Fletcher, "Whither Scientific Deliberation in Health Policy Recommendations? Alice in the Wonderland of Breast Cancer Screening," *New England Journal of Medicine* 336 (1997): 1180–83.

5. See Gina Kolata, "Stand on Mammograms Greeted by Outrage," *New York Times,* January 28, 1997.

6. See Gina Kolata, "Panel Urges Mammograms at 50, Not 40," *New York Times*, November 16, 2009; Gina Kolata, "Mammogram Debate Took Group by Surprise," *New York Times,* November 20, 2009; Kevin Sack, "Screening Debate Reveals Culture Clash in Medicine," *New York Times,* November 20, 2009; and Barbara Ehrenreich, "We Need a New Women's Health Movement," *Los Angeles Times,* December 2, 2009.

7. H. D. Nelson, K. Tyne, A. Naik, et al., "Screening for Breast Cancer: An Update for the U.S. Preventive Services Task Force," *Annals of Internal Medicine* 151 (2009): 727–37.

8. These data come from the National Center for Health Statistics' Multiple Cause-of-Death Public-Use Files. In this case, I use the current ten-year risk of breast cancer death and assume it already reflects the beneficial effect of mammography (in other words, I assume that all American women are currently screened). Inflating the observed rate by 25 percent produces an estimate of what the death rate would be without mammography. (For those wondering why I use 25 percent instead of 20 percent, remember that relative changes are not symmetrical: decreasing 100 by 20 percent produces 80, but 80 must be increased by 25 percent to get back to 100.) The difference in the expected and observed rates is the death benefit. For the general approach, see S. Woloshin, L. M.

Schwartz, and H. G. Welch, "The Risk of Death by Age, Sex, and Smoking Status in the United States: Putting Health Risks in Context," *Journal of the National Cancer Institute* 100 (2008): 845–53.

9.  The simplest way to understand this is to remember that many more women are diagnosed with breast cancer than will ever die of it. Breast cancer incidence is currently about 125 per 100,000; breast cancer mortality is about 25 per 100,000. Let's assume this mortality already includes the beneficial effect of mammography (that is, assume that all American women are currently screened, just as we did above). So the estimated mortality without mammography is 25 percent higher, or 31 per 100,000. So for every 125 diagnosed, about 31 will die and about 94 will not, suggesting about 75 percent (94/125) of women can be equally well treated whether or not they are diagnosed by screening. But let's assume some of the reported incidence represents overdiagnosis *due* to mammography and use one of the higher estimates—30 percent. That means breast cancer incidence without mammography would still be 96 per 100,000. So now for every 96 diagnosed, about 31 will die and about 65 will not. In other words, using even the most conservative assumptions, we see that two-thirds of women can be equally well treated whether or not they are diagnosed by screening.

10. The most recent randomized trial—the Age trial, involving 160,000 forty-year-olds—did show a slightly smaller benefit: about 0.4 per 1,000 women. Despite the tremendous size of the study, the result was not statistically significant, meaning it could be due to chance. See S. M. Moss, H. Cuckle, A. Evans, et al., "Effect of Mammographic Screening from Age 40 Years on Breast Cancer Mortality at 10 Years' Follow-up: A Randomised Controlled Trial," *Lancet* 368 (2006): 2053–60.

11. P. C. Gøtzsche and M. Nielsen, "Screening for Breast Cancer with Mammography," *Cochrane Database of Systematic Reviews* 2009, issue 4, art. no.: CD001877, table 1.15.

12. See Fletcher et al., "Report of the International Workshop."

13. Y. Shen, Y. Yang, L. Y. Inoue, et al., "Role of Detection Method in Predicting Breast Cancer Survival: Analysis of Randomized Screening Trials," *Journal of the National Cancer Institute* 97 (2005): 1195–1203.

14. For the long-term risk of invasive breast cancer developing after a normal mammogram, see E. L. Ashbeck, R. D. Rosenberg, P. M. Stauber, et al., "Benign Breast Biopsy Diagnosis and Subsequent Risk of Breast Cancer," *Cancer Epidemiology, Biomarkers and Prevention* 16 (2007): 467–72. It shows almost the same risk as in the general SEER population (which is remarkable, because New Mexico actually has the lowest risk of breast cancer of all the SEER areas).

15. J. G. Elmore, M. B. Barton, V. M. Moceri, et al., "Ten-year Risk of False Positive Screening Mammograms and Clinical Breast Examinations," *New England Journal of Medicine* 338 (1998): 1089–96.

16. To estimate this, I start with the observation that 60 percent of breast cancers are diagnosed by mammography in the United States; see N. Breen, K. R. Yabroff, and H. I. Meissner, "What Proportion of Breast Cancers Are Detected by Mammography in the United States?" *Cancer Detection and Prevention* 31 (2007): 220–24. The SEER data report that the risk of a fifty-year-old woman developing breast cancer in the next ten years is 24 per 1,000. Using the 60 percent figure, this suggests about 14 cancers per 1,000 are found because of mammography. Since the reduction in death is 1 per 1,000, that leaves 13 per 1,000 for the other two categories. So 13 of 14—or over 90 percent—of

mammographically detected cancers represent either overdiagnosis or early diagnosis with no change in prognosis.

17. C. J. Baines, "Rethinking Breast Screening—Again," *British Medical Journal* 331 (2005): 1031.

18. These data come from seven autopsy studies. Four of the studies involved women who died in the hospital, were not known to have breast cancer, and had previously unsuspected cases diagnosed during the autopsy. Three of the studies were forensic autopsies—consecutive deaths investigated by a coroner (that is, deaths in which homicide was suspected). See H. G. Welch and W. C. Black, "Using Autopsy Series to Estimate the Disease 'Reservoir' for Ductal Carcinoma in Situ of the Breast: How Much More Breast Cancer Can We Find?" *Annals of Internal Medicine* 127 (1997): 1023–28.

19. See P. H. Zahl, "Overdiagnosis of Breast Cancer in Denmark," *British Journal of Cancer* 90 (2004): 1686; E. Paci, J. Warwick, P. Falini, et al., "Overdiagnosis in Screening: Is the Increase in Breast Cancer Incidence Rates a Cause for Concern?" *Journal of Medical Screening* 11 (2004): 23–27; P. H. Zahl, B. H. Strand, and J. Mæhlen, "Breast Cancer Incidence in Norway and Sweden during Introduction of Nation-wide Screening: Prospective Cohort Study," *British Medical Journal* 328 (2004): 921–24; IARC Handbooks of Cancer Prevention, vol. 7: *Breast Cancer Screening* (Lyon, France: International Agency for Research on Cancer Press, 2002), 147.

20. This is because screening a previously unscreened population detects so-called prevalent cancers—those that have not yet presented clinically. To understand this, first assume that all breast cancers progress to cause symptoms or death—that is, there is no overdiagnosis. Now imagine that mammography typically advances the time of cancer diagnosis by two years (called the lead time). Now imagine starting a national screening program: there is two years' worth of impending cancer out there that you will detect very quickly. So even if there is no overdiagnosis, the incidence of cancer must temporarily rise. In fact, this must happen for screening to help people (or else no one is being detected early).

21. K. J. Jørgensen and P. C. Gøtzsche, "Overdiagnosis in Publicly Organised Mammography Screening Programmes: Systematic Review of Incidence Trends," *British Medical Journal* 339 (2009): b2587.

22. P. H. Zahl, J. Mæhlen, and H. G. Welch, "The Natural History of Invasive Breast Cancers Detected by Screening Mammography," *Archives of Internal Medicine* 168 (2008): 2311–16.

23. To get a flavor of what researchers were thinking in this period, see S. E. King and D. Schottenfeld, "The 'Epidemic' of Breast Cancer in the U.S.—Determining the Factors," *Oncology* 10 (1996): 453–62; J. M. Liff, J. F. Sung, W. H. Chow, et al., "Does Increased Detection Account for the Rising Incidence of Breast Cancer?" *American Journal of Public Health* 81 (1991): 462–65; L. Garfinkel, C. C. Boring, and C. W. Heath Jr., "Changing Trends. An Overview of Breast Cancer Incidence and Mortality," *Cancer* 74 (1994): 222–27; M. S. Simon, D. Lemanne, A. G. Schwartz, et al., "Recent Trends in the Incidence of In Situ and Invasive Breast Cancer in the Detroit Metropolitan Area (1975–1988)," *Cancer* 71 (1993): 769–74.

24. The one-third estimate comes from D. Page, W. Dupont, L. Rogers, et al., "Continued Local Recurrence of Carcinoma 15–25 Years after a Diagnosis of Low-grade Ductal Carcinoma In Situ of the Breast Treated Only by Biopsy," *Cancer* 76 (1995): 1197–2000. But based on Dr. Black's and my review of autopsy studies and the work of others—see V. L.

Ernster, J. Barclay, K. Kerlikowske, et al., "Incidence of and Treatment for Ductal Carcinoma In Situ of the Breast," *Journal of the American Medical Association* 275 (1996): 913–18—it seems clear this is a high estimate.

25. P. H. Zahl et al., "Natural History."

26. See S. Zackrisson, I. Andersson, L. Janzon, et al., "Rate of Over-diagnosis of Breast Cancer 15 Years after End of Malmö Mammographic Screening Trial: Follow-up Study," *British Medical Journal* 332 (2006): 689–92; and P. Gøtzsche, O. Hartling, M. Nielsen, et al., "Breast Screening: The Facts—or Maybe Not," *British Medical Journal* 338 (2009): b86.

27. K. Jørgensen and P. Gøtzsche, "Content of Invitations for Publicly Funded Screening Mammography," *British Medical Journal* 332 (2006): 538–41.

28. H. G. Welch, S. Woloshin, and L. M. Schwartz, "The Sea of Uncertainty Surrounding Ductal Carcinoma In Situ—the Price of Screening Mammography," *Journal of the National Cancer Institute* 100 (2008): 228–29.

## CHAPTER 7: WE STUMBLE ONTO INCIDENTALOMAS THAT MIGHT BE CANCER

1. J. R. Jett, "Limitations of Screening for Lung Cancer with Low-dose Spiral Computed Tomography," *Clinical Cancer Research* 11 (2005): 4988s–92s.

2. You might reasonably wonder why, given the whole-body CT scanning data presented in chapter 3 (showing 86 percent of healthy patients had at least one abnormality), this estimate isn't higher. The reason is twofold: (1) most CT scans are not so extensive (that is, they are limited to one portion of the body), and (2) not every abnormality constitutes an incidentaloma.

3. M. K. Gould, J. Fletcher, M. D. Iannettoni, et al., "Evaluation of Patients with Pulmonary Nodules: When Is It Lung Cancer? ACCP Evidence-based Clinical Practice Guidelines (second edition)," *Chest* 132 (2007): 108s–30s.

4. See R. P. Myers, A. Fong, and A. A. Shaheen, "Utilization Rates, Complications and Costs of Percutaneous Liver Biopsy: A Population-based Study Including 4275 Biopsies," *Liver International* 28 (2008): 705–12.

5. J. Graunt, "Foundations of Vital Statistics," in J. R. Newman, ed., *The World of Mathematics*, vol. 3 (Redmond, WA: Tempus Books, 1988), 1399–1413.

6. Of course, they will also vary by gender. But since the data on the prevalence of incidentalomas were not stratified by gender and typically involved people in their early fifties, I chose to use the risk of death for fifty-year-olds of both sexes.

7. The data here come from the sources listed in the two references below, with the exception of the prevalence of thyroid nodules by ultrasound; for that data, see S. Ezzat, D. A. Sarti, D. R. Cain, et al., "Thyroid Incidentalomas: Prevalence by Palpation and Ultrasonography," *Archives of Internal Medicine* 154 (1994): 1838–40. The division (and subtraction) is my own doing. . . .

8. Their average age was fifty-four, two-thirds were male, and all were able to afford the approximately $1,000 charge (not covered by insurance). See C. D. Furtado, D. A. Aguirre, C. B. Sirlin, et al., "Whole-body CT Screening: Spectrum of Findings and Recommendations in 1192 Patients," *Radiology* 237 (2005): 385–94. The data on nodules in smokers comes from the Mayo Clinic. See S. J. Swensen, J. R. Jett, J. A. Sloan, et al., "Screening for Lung Cancer with Low-dose Spiral Computed Tomography," *American Journal of Respiratory Critical Care Medicine* 165 (2002): 508–13.

9. You can obtain the risk of dying from a specific cancer between any two specified ages (in this case ages fifty and sixty) at the SEER Web site, http://seer.cancer.gov/faststats/selections.php?series=cancer.

The risk of lung cancer death stratified by smoking status comes from our paper, S. Woloshin, L. M. Schwartz, and H. G. Welch, "The Risk of Death by Age, Sex, and Smoking Status in the United States: Putting Health Risks in Context," *Journal of the National Cancer Institute* 100 (2008): 845–53.

10. Note that if one chose to use a twenty-year time frame, the chance for intervening abnormalities to be responsible for a death twenty years later only gets greater, making these overestimates even larger.

11. E. V. Finlayson and J. D. Birkmeyer, "Operative Mortality with Elective Surgery in Older Adults," *Effective Clinical Practice* 4 (2001): 172–77.

12. Each tumor was measured at least two times (about three months apart) before it was removed. See J. Zhang, S. K. Kang, L. Wang, et al., "Distribution of Renal Tumor Growth Rates Determined by Using Serial Volumetric CT Measurements," *Radiology* 250 (2009): 137–44. Note the article reports volumetric doubling times. Because volumes rise with the cube of the dimension, a two-year volume-doubling time translates into a six-year dimension-doubling time, during which the volume has increased eightfold ($2^3$).

13. See the American Urological Association guidelines "Management of the Clinical Stage 1 Renal Mass" (2009) at http://www.auanet.org/content/guidelines-and-quality-care/clinical-guidelines/main-reports/renalmass09.pdf.

14. Then again, some patients might want to be involved in this kind of decision. Although the issue is complex, a doctor can express this tension before the scan is taken. He or she could say something like, "If we find an abnormality that we don't know what to do with, would you like to be informed about it and possibly worry about it, or would you rather not know?" Yes, it's clunky, but this is one case where ignorance really may be bliss.

Another way to deal with the situation is by obtaining "community informed consent"; see L. Irwig and P. Glasziou, "Informed Consent for Screening by Community Sampling," *Effective Clinical Practice* 3 (2000): 47–50. The idea starts by acknowledging that the ideal—ensuring that before conducting any testing, patients are fully informed about the pros and cons of acting on or ignoring incidentalomas—is simply impractical. There is just not enough time. But it would be possible to focus attention on educating representative samples of the population and then having them vote on what to do. If the informed community sample voted that, on balance, learning about and pursuing a category of incidentalomas was undesirable, radiologists would not report them. If they decided that learning about and pursuing another category of incidentalomas was desirable, radiologists would routinely report them.

15. D. Ost, A. M. Fein, and S. H. Feinsilver, "Clinical Practice. The Solitary Pulmonary Nodule," *New England Journal of Medicine* 348 (2003): 2535–42.

16. W. C. Black, "Lung Cancer," in B. S. Kramer, J. K. Gohagan, and P. C. Prorok, eds., *Cancer Screening: Theory and Practice* (New York: Marcel Dekker, 1999).

17. See C. Henschke, D. McCauley, D. Yankelevitz, et al., "Early Lung Cancer Action Project: Overall Design and Findings from Baseline Screening," *Lancet* 354 (1999): 99–105; M. A. Jewett and A. Zuniga, "Renal Tumor Natural History: The Rationale and Role for Active Surveillance," *Urologic Clinics of North America* 35 (2008): 627–34; and S. G. Silverman, B. Y. Lee, S. E. Seltzer, et al., "Small (< or = 3 cm) Renal Masses: Correlation of Spiral CT Features and Pathologic Findings," *American Journal of Roentgenology* 163 (1994): 597–605.

CHAPTER 8: WE LOOK HARDER FOR EVERYTHING ELSE

1.  See the Cardiac Arrhythmia Suppression Trial investigators, "Preliminary Report: Effect of Encainide and Flecainide on Mortality in a Randomized Trial of Arrhythmia Suppression after Myocardial Infarction," *New England Journal of Medicine* 321 (1989): 406–12; and H. L. Greene, D. M. Roden, R. J. Katz, et al., "The Cardiac Arrhythmia Suppression Trial: First CAST . . . then CAST-II," *Journal of the American College of Cardiology* 19 (1992): 894–98.

2.  See D. C. Dyson, K. H. Danbe, J. A. Bamber, et al., "Monitoring Women at Risk for Preterm Labor," *New England Journal of Medicine* 338 (1998): 15–19. The study also included a third arm that was in between the two described here—women who had daily nurse contact but no home monitoring. This also had no effect on the rate of premature birth and it had an intermediate effect on visits and drug treatment.

3.  Z. Alfirevic, D. Devane, and G. M. Gyte, "Continuous Cardiotocography (CTG) as a Form of Electronic Fetal Monitoring (EFM) for Fetal Assessment during Labour," *Cochrane Database of Systematic Reviews* 3 (2006): CD006066; see http://mrw .interscience.wiley.com/cochrane/clsysrev/articles/CD006066/frame.html.

4.  This calculation depends on three inputs: (1) the 66 percent increase in C-section rates caused by monitoring, (2) the overall rate of C-sections in the United States (which was 310 per 1,000 births in 2006; see below), and (3) the frequency with which intrauterine electronic fetal monitoring is used in the United States (which was estimated at 83 percent of all births in 1997, see below). There is only one possible set of numbers for the frequency of C-section with and without monitoring that will have a ratio of 1.66 (that's the 66 percent increase) and will produce a weighted average of 310 per 1,000 (where the weight is .83 for monitoring and .17 for no monitoring): 330 and 200 per 1,000.

    The overall rate of C-section in the United States comes from B. E. Hamilton, J. A. Martin, and S. J. Ventura, "Births: Preliminary Data for 2006," *National Vital Statistics Reports*, vol. 56, no. 7 (Hyattsville, MD: National Center for Health Statistics, 2007). See http://www.cdc.gov/nchs/data/nvsr/nvsr56/nvsr56_07.pdf.

    The frequency of monitoring comes from S. C. Curtin and M. M. Park, "Trends in the Attendant, Place, and Timing of Births, and in the Use of Obstetric Interventions: United States, 1989–97," *National Vital Statistics Reports*, vol. 47, no. 27 (Hyattsville, MD: National Center for Health Statistics, 1999). See http://www.cdc.gov/nchs/data/nvsr/ nvsr47/nvs47_27.pdf.

5.  See http://www.ahrq.gov/clinic/uspstf/uspsiefm.htm.

6.  Curtin and Park, "Trends."

7.  Given the absence of good utilization data, you might reasonably wonder how I can confidently say this. First, it is what the obstetricians themselves say; see J. T. Parer, "Obstetric Technologies: What Determines Clinical Acceptance or Rejection of Results of Randomized Controlled Trials?" *American Journal of Obstetrics and Gynecology* 188 (2003): 1622–25. Second, the above federal survey of new mothers suggests that 83 percent of births are monitored and 64 percent of women have at least one ultrasound during the pregnancy (they do not report on home uterine monitoring). Finally, it is also the judgment of the U.S. Preventive Services Task Force. They wrote that "home uterine monitoring is no longer considered a part of standard obstetrical care" and that despite their recommendations to the contrary, both fetal monitoring and obstetrical ultrasounds have "become common practice in the U.S."

8. R. A. Filly, "Obstetrical Sonography: The Best Way to Terrify a Pregnant Woman," *Journal of Ultrasound in Medicine* 19 (2000): 1–5.

9. T. J. Hassold and P. A. Jacobs, "Trisomy in Man," *Annual Review of Genetics* 18 (1984): 69–97.

10. In case the calculation is not obvious from the text, let me explicitly work through it here. The probability that a detected abnormality reflects disease is directly related to how common the disease is (in this case, 3 per 1,000) and inversely related to how common the abnormality is (in this case, 100 per 1,000). In decimal form the numbers are .003/.1 = .03, or 3 percent. In other words 3 percent of detected abnormalities represent trisomy. The remaining 97 percent do not. (Note: This calculation assumes that every fetus with trisomy has one of the anatomic abnormalities, which is undoubtedly not true. If I accounted for this it would only increase the estimate of overdiagnosis.)

11. A. Ghidini, "Amniocentesis: Technique and Complications," in D. S. Basow, ed., *UpToDate* (Waltham, MA: UpToDate, 2009).

12. R. Smith-Bindman, W. Hosmer, V. A. Feldstein, et al., "Second-trimester Ultrasound to Detect Fetuses with Down Syndrome: A Meta-analysis," *Journal of the American Medical Association* 285 (2001): 1044–55.

13. Natalie Angier, "Ultrasound and Fury: One Mother's Ordeal," *New York Times,* November 26, 1996, http://query.nytimes.com/gst/fullpage.html?res=9E07E2D9103DF935A157 52C1A960958260&sec=&spon=.

14. See http://www.cochrane.org/reviews/en/ab001451.html and http://www.cochrane.org/reviews/en/ab000182.html.

15. See http://www.ahrq.gov/clinic/uspstf/uspspg.htm.

16. These data come from the evidence synthesis done by the U.S. Preventive Services Task Force. The synthesis includes data from four randomized trials of AAA screening. See http://www.ncbi.nlm.nih.gov/books/bv.fcgi?rid=hstat3.table.30132. The numbers in the table presented here have all been converted into a single metric: the risk of the event over five years.

17. Note: Although the task force makes no recommendation for never-smokers and recommends a one-time screen for smokers age sixty-five to seventy-five, these data reflect all men—smokers and nonsmokers—over sixty-five who were included in the major randomized trials. The panel was forced to make an estimate that the benefit would be greater for smokers.

## CHAPTER 9: WE CONFUSE DNA WITH DISEASE

1. My twenty-year-old daughter (who kindly reviewed this chapter) thought another sentence was warranted at this point. Something like, "Needless to say, I did not have my first girlfriend until I was twenty-five."

2. Fiscal Year 1999 President's Budget Request; statement by Dr. Francis S. Collins, director, National Human Genome Research Institute, before the House Subcommittee on Labor, Health and Human Services, Education and Related Agencies, March 12, 1998.

3. To learn how we can get confused on this point in clinical medicine, see More Depth: Phenotype, Genotype, and Blood Clots, at www.beacon.org/overdiagnosed.

4. Even with a straightforward case like cystic fibrosis, however, disease development is somewhat more complicated than this explanation. It turns out that there is more than

one genetic mutation that leads to cystic fibrosis, and some mutations lead to more severe disease than others (and the effect of some mutations is even modified by environmental factors). So while the penetrance of the so-called severe genotypes is virtually 100 percent for pancreatic insufficiency (which inhibits digestion), penetrance can be lower for other problems, such as meconium ileus (or intestinal obstruction), liver disease, and diabetes. See R. Dorfman and J. Zielenski, "Genotype-Phenotype Correlations in Cystic Fibrosis," in A. Bush, E. W. F. W. Alton, J. C. Davies, et al., eds., *Cystic Fibrosis in the 21st Century* (Basel, Switzerland: S. Karger, AG, 2006), 61–68.

5.  See S. Chen and G. Parmigiani, "Meta-analysis of BRCA1 and BRCA2 Penetrance," *Journal of Clinical Oncology* 25 (2007): 1329–33.

6.  See J. Peto, N. Collins, R. Barfoot, et al., "Prevalence of BRCA1 and BRCA2 Gene Mutations in Patients with Early-onset Breast Cancer," *Journal of the National Cancer Institute* 91 (1999): 943–49.

7.  There are a number of risk factors that have been associated with increased breast cancer risk, including older age, family history, early age of menarche, no children, and late age of first childbirth. If you are interested in calculating your own risk, go to http://www.cancer.gov/bcrisktool/.

8.  The situation is even muddier than I have described. The phrase *disease gene* often appears in the general press (as in the *breast cancer gene*), which is why I use it here. But geneticists would prefer that the term not be used. They point out that the word *gene* should refer to a section of DNA that codes for a specific protein. There aren't genes for disease, per se; instead, there are changes in the DNA sequence of a gene that can lead to disease. Such changes could be labeled *mutations* or *variants,* and while both words mean the same thing, the former feels more severe and there is an increasing tendency to stay away from it. A more direct approach might be to use *disease genotype* for a highly penetrant mutation/variant and a *susceptibility genotype* for a less penetrant one. Getting the language right is tough stuff. . . .

9.  See D. H. Andersen, "Cystic Fibrosis of the Pancreas and Its Relation to Celiac Disease: A Clinical and Pathological Study," *American Journal of Diseases of Children* 56 (1938): 344–99; and G. Huntington, "On Chorea," *Medical and Surgical Reporter: A Weekly Journal* 26 (1872): 317–21 (available at http://en.wikisource.org/wiki/On_Chorea).

10. At the same time, I believe a little controlled bloodletting is a good thing for the well. I like to think it gives the body a little practice in responding to blood loss, both in shifting fluids to maintain blood pressure and in making extra new cells. Doing it is easy, doesn't cost anything, and you get free food. All you need to do is donate during your local blood drive.

11. If you lose a moderate amount of blood and don't have hemochromatosis, you will become iron deficient. That will impair your ability to make red blood cells, and you will develop what is called an iron deficiency anemia. To avoid this, patients who have experienced a moderate blood loss are typically given iron supplements.

12. A. Pietrangelo, "Hereditary Hemochromatosis—A New Look at an Old Disease," *New England Journal of Medicine* 350 (2004): 2383–97.

13. E. P. Whitlock, B. A. Garlitz, E. L. Harris, et al., "Screening for Hereditary Hemochromatosis: A Systematic Review for the U.S. Preventive Services Task Force," *Annals of Internal Medicine* 145 (2006): 209–23.

14. For more on snips, see http://www.ncbi.nlm.nih.gov/About/primer/snps.html.

15. S. L. Zheng, J. Sun, F. Wiklund, et al., "Cumulative Association of Five Genetic Variants with Prostate Cancer," *New England Journal of Medicine* 358 (2008): 910–19.

16. The questions I raise here about this genetic test for prostate cancer first appeared in an essay I wrote for the *Washington Post*; see H. G. Welch, "A Test You Shouldn't Jump At: A Genetic Test for Prostate Cancer May Boost Worry, Little More," *Washington Post*, February 19, 2008.

17. There is some uncertainty about both the effect of removing the ovaries on cardiovascular risk and the value of starting estrogen in this setting. See R. A. Lobo, "Surgical Menopause and Cardiovascular Risks," *Menopause* 14 (2007): 562–66. There is little uncertainty that some doctors would make these suggestions.

18. H. H. Heng, "Cancer Genome Sequencing: The Challenges Ahead," *BioEssays* 29 (2007): 783–94.

19. In fact, it has already happened. It's called preimplantation genetic diagnosis (PGD), and it's often used by parents who carry a genetic trait for a particular disease. The embryos are fertilized in a laboratory using the sperm from the father and the eggs from the mother. Each embryo receives genetic screening, and only the embryos without the defective gene are implanted in the mother. In other words, it's genetic selection.

    It's an approach that has been used to select children who are free of cystic fibrosis, a disease that becomes apparent early in life. But recently, in the United Kingdom, it was used to select for the absence of BRCA1—the so-called breast cancer gene. It's an aggressive form of screening, to be sure. And the unfortunate truth is that despite testing, girls born via PGD who don't carry the BRCA1 gene remain at about average risk for breast cancer.

CHAPTER 10: GET THE FACTS

1. http://www.thyroidawareness.com/cancer.php (last accessed March 5, 2009).

2. As with all cancer incidence and mortality statistics presented in this book, these data come from the National Cancer Institute's Surveillance Epidemiology and End Results (SEER) program, http://seer.cancer.gov/statistics/.

3. This story is a collage of patient stories obtained on the Web. All the quotes are real.

4. http://www.sciencedaily.com/releases/2008/04/080421180946.htm (last accessed March 5, 2009).

5. To understand why survival always exaggerates the effectiveness of early diagnosis, let's return to the simplified example of lead-time bias. But now assume that mammography does help women live longer—that is, death *is* delayed. Without screening, women live four years (diagnosed at age eighty-six, death at ninety). Imagine that screening extended their lives by one year (death at age ninety-one). But because screening also advanced the time of diagnosis (from eighty-six to eighty-four), screened women now appear to live seven years (diagnosed at age eighty-four, death at ninety-one). That's an apparent benefit of three years, while the actual benefit is one year.

    Even more worrisome is that these biases can obscure a harmful effect of screening. If screened women died one year earlier (at eighty-nine), they would still appear to live one year longer than those not screened: five years (diagnosed at age eighty-four, death at eighty-nine) versus four years (diagnosed at age eighty-six, death at ninety).

6. In fact, the measure need not be of survival. It could be about the proportion that avoids any one outcome (death, heart attack, amputation, or hip fracture) over any fixed time

(two, five, ten, or seven and a half years). Consider the outcome of avoiding an amputation in a population of diabetics. I am confident that a group of diabetics diagnosed early (say, using a blood sugar of greater than 126 as the cutoff) will have a higher amputation-free survival at five years than a group of diabetics diagnosed later (say, using a blood sugar of greater than 140 as the cutoff). That does not mean that early detection necessarily helped anyone; it means only that people with milder disease are more likely to do well regardless.

7.   The other reason may be that it is easier to understand relative risks. People are just more familiar with statements like "a 10 percent increase" and "a 30 percent reduction." Conveying the underlying absolute risks is more complex: it requires more numbers (because there are two absolute risks underlying each relative risk); these numbers are often very small (decimals are often needed, or the numbers have to be expressed per 1,000 or per 10,000 people); and a complete statement requires a time frame (for example, per year or over ten years).

8.   As you might imagine, I'm rounding here to make the math easy. The relative risk reduction estimated by the U.S. Preventive Services Task Force in its meta-analysis of all nine trials is 16 percent. See "Effectiveness of Mammography in Reducing Breast Cancer Mortality" at http://www.ahrq.gov/clinic/3rduspstf/breastcancer/bcscrnsum1.htm#results.

9.   Again, I'm rounding. The actual estimate by the U.S. Preventive Services Task Force is that 1,224 women need to be screened for an average of fourteen years for one to benefit.

10.  P. C. Gøtzsche, O. J. Hartling, M. Nielsen, et al., "Breast Screening: The Facts—or Maybe Not," *British Medical Journal* 338 (2009): b86.

11.  J. G. Elmore, M. B. Barton, V. M. Moceri, et al., "Ten-year Risk of False Positive Screening Mammograms and Clinical Breast Examinations," *New England Journal of Medicine* 338 (1998): 1089–96.

12.  Allow me to explain the number first and then I will move on to its source. As I said earlier, a mammographically detected cancer can fall into one of three buckets: (1) an overdiagnosed cancer (one not destined to cause symptoms or death); (2) a clinically significant cancer for which early detection alters the prognosis (that's the death benefit); and (3) a clinically significant cancer for which early detection *does not* alter the prognosis (the patient can be cured of her disease regardless of whether it is detected clinically or by screening, or the patient is destined to die from her disease regardless of whether it is detected clinically or by screening). This number reflects this third category.

Now let me address where the number comes from. It is actually harder to estimate than it should be. Conceptually, it is just the rate of mammographic breast cancer detection after subtracting the number of women who experienced the death benefit (about 1 per 1,000) and the number of women who were overdiagnosed (2 to 10 per 1,000). To estimate this, I start with the observation that 60 percent of breast cancers are diagnosed by mammography in the United States (see N. Breen, K. R. Yabroff, and H. I. Meissner, "What Proportion of Breast Cancers Are Detected by Mammography in the United States?" *Cancer Detection and Prevention* 31 (2007): 220–24). The SEER data report that the risk for a fifty-year-old to develop breast cancer in the next ten years is 24 per 1,000; that suggests about 14 per 1,000 are found by screening mammography. Subtracting out the death benefit and overdiagnosis, that leaves 3 to 11 per 1,000 women in whom the time of diagnosis was advanced but no benefit occurred. Using data from the randomized trials that include detection rates produces slightly higher numbers, which would be expected, given that the SEER data do not reflect complete penetration of mammography. To convey this effect and a sense of uncertainty, I use 5 to 15 per 1,000 here.

13. See "Breast Cancer Screening Peril—Negative Consequences of the Breast Screening Programme," *London Times,* February 19, 2009, http://www.timesonline.co.uk/tol/ comment/letters/article5761650.ece; and C. Smyth, "NHS Rips Up Breast Cancer Leaflet and Starts All Over Again," *London Times,* February 21, 2009, http://www.timesonline .co.uk/tol/life_and_style/health/article5776804.ece.

## CHAPTER 11: GET THE SYSTEM

1. R. M. Neer, C. D. Arnaud, J. R. Zanchetta, et al., "Effect of Parathyroid Hormone (1–34) on Fractures and Bone Mineral Density in Postmenopausal Women with Osteoporosis," *New England Journal of Medicine* 344 (2001): 1434–41.

2. Although the drug-company study referenced above collected data on both symptomatic and asymptomatic compression fractures, the publication only reported on the combination.

3. I feel compelled to add that some of my ancestors were serious capitalists. My great-great-grandfather started a bank in the mid-nineteenth century and helped the federal government finance the Civil War. His offspring managed it over the next century.

4. The *invisible hand* is the term economists use to describe the self-regulating nature of markets to produce socially useful results. Although attributed to Adam Smith and his book *The Wealth of Nations* (published around the time of the American Revolution), he actually used the term only three times.

5. This is one of many ways to express the conditions required for a perfect market and is not intended to be a complete list. Instead I have focused on the conditions in medical care that clearly violate the perfect-market conditions. The most basic condition for a perfect market is often not even mentioned: markets are vehicles to price tradable goods, so to have a market, consumers must know and pay that price (the first two prerequisites on my list). The most common conditions for perfect markets enumerated by economists are perfect information and rationality (the second two prerequisites on my list). In addition, there is the condition of perfect competition: that buyers and sellers are price takers and cannot influence demand (my final prerequisite). Other conditions for a perfect market not listed here include no barriers to market entry (clearly violated, given the long training period required for doctors), no externalities or public goods, and no information costs.

6. See Maryann Napoli, "PSA Screening Test for Prostate Cancer: An Interview with Otis Brawley, MD," May 2003, http://medicalconsumers.org/2003/05/01/psa-screening-test -for-prostate-cancer/.

7. Probably one of the most important voices taking issue with the growing commercialization of medicine has been that of Arnold Relman. Dr. Relman was the editor of the *New England Journal of Medicine* in 1980 when he coined the term *medical-industrial complex.* His book *A Second Opinion* (New York: PublicAffairs, 2007) succinctly makes the case for why medicine's transformation from a professional enterprise to a business has been a disaster. It's a good read.

8.  H. G. Welch, "Campaign Myths: Prevention as Cure All," *New York Times,* October 7, 2008.

9.  This is according to OpenSecrets.org, which lists health professionals as the fifth-largest donor to members of Congress, pharmaceuticals as the seventeenth, hospitals/nursing homes as the twenty-first, and health services as the fortieth. Put them all together and medical care is the third-largest contributor, behind retirees and lawyers. See http://www.opensecrets.org/industries/mems.php.

10. Gina Kolata, "Forty Years' War: Grant System Leads Cancer Researchers to Play It Safe," *New York Times,* June 27, 2009, http://www.nytimes.com/2009/06/28/health/research/28cancer.html?_r=1.

11. F. B. Palumbo and C. D. Mullins, "The Development of Direct-to-Consumer Prescription Drug Advertising Regulation," *Food and Drug Law Journal* 57 (2002): 423–43.

12. H. Moses, E. R. Dorsey, D. H. Matheson, et al., "Financial Anatomy of Biomedical Research," *Journal of the American Medical Association* 294 (2005): 1333–42.

13. A. H. Krist, S. H. Woolf, and R. E. Johnson, "How Physicians Approach Prostate Cancer Screening Before and After Losing a Lawsuit," *Annals of Family Medicine* 5 (2007): 120–25.

14. This estimate assumes a 20 percent mortality reduction from screening. In other words, without screening, five women die from metastatic breast cancer; with screening, four women die from metastatic breast cancer. If each of the five made the typical plaintiff's case that screening would have saved her life, only one would have been right.

## CHAPTER 12: GET THE BIG PICTURE

1.  To construct figure 12.1, I had to choose how harm related to the spectrum of abnormality. Given that it might have either a slightly positive or a slightly negative slope, I chose a flat line. Had I chosen a line with a slightly positive slope (more severe abnormality, more harm—as in the surgery example), the area of net harm in figure 12.2 would appear smaller. Had I chosen a line with a slightly negative slope (more severe abnormality, less harm—as in the hypertension example), the area of net harm would appear larger.

2.  Remember that while a small, short study can demonstrate a big effect (the VA cooperative study of severe hypertension needed to follow only a hundred and fifty patients for a year and a half), it takes a big, long study to demonstrate a small effect (the typical randomized trial of mammography studied fifty thousand women for a decade or more). Studies of intervention in low-risk people necessarily mean that investigators are looking for small effects. So they require big, long studies—some so big and so long that they could never be done.

3.  A positive-feedback loop occurs when a system responds to disturbance in the same direction as the disturbance—that is, the system speeds the process. The perturbation becomes self-reinforcing. In this case, more diagnosis begets more diagnosis.

4.  See http://www.roadtoearlydetection.org/educate.shtml.

5.  A. E. Raffle and J. A. Muir Gray, eds., *Screening: Evidence and Practice* (New York: Oxford University Press, 2007).

6.  E. Silverman, S. Woloshin, L. M. Schwartz, et al., "Women's Views on Breast Cancer Risk and Screening Mammography: A Qualitative Interview Study," *Medical Decision Making* 21 (2001): 231–40.

7.  See chapter 2 of my book *Should I Be Tested for Cancer?* (Berkeley: University of California Press, 2004) for a full discussion of false-positive results in cancer screening.
8.  L. M. Schwartz, S. Woloshin, F. J. Fowler Jr., and H. G. Welch, "Enthusiasm for Cancer Screening in the United States," *Journal of the American Medical Association* 291 (2004): 71–78.
9.  C. Lerman, B. Trock, B. K. Rimer, et al., "Psychological and Behavioral Implications of Abnormal Mammograms," *Annals of Internal Medicine* 114 (1991): 657–61.
10. It's been called the "popularity paradox of screening." Raffle and Muir Gray, eds., *Screening,* 68.
11. These two self-reinforcing cycles may explain why both doctors and their patients are reluctant to do less cervical cancer screening. See K. R. Yabroff, M. Saraiya, H. I. Meissner, et al., "Specialty Differences in Primary Care Physician Reports of Papanicolaou Test Screening Practices: A National Survey, 2006 to 2007," *Annals of Internal Medicine* 151 (2009): 602–11; and B. E. Sirovich, S. Woloshin, and L. M. Schwartz, "Screening for Cervical Cancer: Will Women Accept Less?" *American Journal of Medicine* 118 (2005): 151–58.
12. Guy Gugliotta, "One Researcher's Plan: Fight Storms with Storms," *Washington Post,* October 3, 2005.

## CONCLUSION

1.  This quote is taken from a book by David Alt titled *Glacial Lake Missoula and Its Humongous Floods* (Missoula, MT: Mountain Press Publishing Company, 2001). It's a great introduction to this fascinating cataclysmic geologic event.
2.  Including in Yellowstone itself. During the last ice age, the Yellowstone plateau had its own ice sheet (distinct from the continental ice sheet). Glaciers from this ice sheet formed ice dams on the Lamar River; the dams subsequently failed and released massive floods in the Paradise Valley.
3.  See Nancy Cordes, "Mammogram Task Force Goes before Congress," CBS News, December 2, 2009, http://www.cbsnews.com/stories/2009/12/02/eveningnews/main5868631 .shtml?tag=contentMain;content; and Robert Pear and David Herszenhorn, "Senate Backs Preventive Health Care for Women," *New York Times,* December 4, 2009, http://query.nytimes.com/gst/fullpage.html?res=9F02E6DD113FF937A35751C1A96F9C8B63.
4.  Keep in mind that the definition of *symptoms* is slippery. Ordinary experiences are increasingly being redefined as symptoms. Here there is no dire outcome on the horizon.
5.  Like most general rules, there are exceptions. Symptom improvement is not a foolproof test of benefit for two reasons. First, some people feel better just because they do something. That is the placebo effect: people sometimes experience a benefit even when they take an inert sugar pill or when they receive a faked surgery. Second, some symptoms, by their very nature, wax and wane spontaneously. People with back pain know this quite well; on some days, their backs feel great, on other days, they feel awful.

    These two factors can lead people to judge an intervention as beneficial when in fact what is really happening is either a placebo effect or a spontaneous improvement. Consequently, the most trustworthy test of an intervention for current symptoms is still a randomized trial—a true experiment in which people are randomly given the drug or a placebo and then undergo a standardized symptom assessment. If the drug works, then the people randomized to get the drug will do better, on average, than those randomized to placebo.

6.  Again, as for most general rules, there are exceptions. Some symptoms are better off left alone, particularly when they don't bother people very much. And since some symptoms go away on their own, there is no reason to deal with them early.

7.  My father died of metastatic colon cancer at age sixty. Even though I know this is a relatively weak risk factor for colon cancer, it was enough to make me choose to have a screening colonoscopy at age fifty. I'm not sure whether I will do so again (my hesitancy has nothing to do with my testing experience, which was uneventful—in fact, I found it interesting).

8.  At this point, our only way of knowing if a person was overdiagnosed is if that person got diagnosed, never got treated, and eventually died without ever having developed problems from the disease in question.

abdominal aortic aneurysm: anxiety from diagnosis, 115; defined, 39; increase in diagnosis, 41; overdiagnosis of, 41, 44, 115; risk factors, 40; risk of rupture, 39; screening for, 113–14, 147, 186, 210n16; spectrum of abnormality in, 40

Ablin, Professor Richard J., 60

abnormality: ambiguous, 34–35; and apparent improvement in outcome, 174–75; and apparent increase in prevalence, 41–42, 174–75; commonality of, xi, 36, 38, 43–44, 101, 103, 108; defined, xvi; detection of, that may never bother us, xii, xiv, 9–10, 32, 44, 54–55, 61, 190; detection of, which have nothing to do with symptoms, 43, 91–92, 164–65; expansion of definition, xv, 167, 171–78; mild, 8–9, 13, 18, 20–24, 26, 28, 41, 83, 175; numerical, 2, 15, 20–23, 27, 31–32, 52, 167, 171; overdiagnosis of, 10, 100, 190, 199n22; overstating the value of treating, 27; reservoir of, 35–38, 49, 94; screening for, 102–3; structural, 167; unexpected, 34–35, 91–92, 119, 157. *See also* numeric rules; spectrum of abnormality

advertising, 159

Africa, 179

Air Force / Texas Coronary Atherosclerosis Prevention Study, 21, 25

Alamaro, Moshe, 178–79

Alaska, 32

Alaska Area Native Health Service, 33

American Academy of Pediatrics, 28

American Cancer Society, 58, 74, 75, 81, 85, 156

American College of Obstetricians and Gynecologists, 70

American Diabetes Association, 28

American Institute of Ultrasound in Medicine, 107

American Society of Endocrinologists, 138, 140

amniocentesis, 108–10; induced miscarriages, 108

amputation, 15, 17

anencephaly, 110

Angier, Natalie, 110–12, 168

angina, 21

Anglican mission hospital, 33

antibiotics, 34

Apgar scores, 105

appendicitis, 92

Apple Computer Company, 153

Aquarius Plateau, 39

arthritis, 36; rheumatoid, 29

arthroscopic surgery, 37

aspirin, 2

atherosclerosis, 113

Atlantic Ocean, 179

autopsy, 96; studies, 63, 65, 82

Aventis Pharmaceuticals, 24

baby boomers, xii

bad event: defined, 9; prevention, 15–16; probability of, 6–9, 12–13

benefit of treatment, 5–9, 20–22, 24, 26–28, 30, 152; declining with milder abnormalities, 8–10, 13, 18, 20–22, 24, 26, 28, 42, 78, 175; increasing with severe abnormalities, 10, 19; measures of, 8, 174; net benefit, 172–74; no benefit, 14, 16, 30, 43–44, 64; potential benefit, 13, 18, 25, 45, 59, 170–74, 183; across the spectrum of abnormality, 8–10, 14, 172–74

Bering Sea, 33

Bethel, Alaska, 33

bilirubin, 188
biopsy, 72, 75, 90; brain, 177; breast, 75, 81, 89, 119, 149; of incidentaloma, 93–94; lung, 69, 99; for melanoma, 65–66; prostate, xi, 46–52, 58–61; risks of, 81, 94; saturation, 49; thyroid, 62–63, 139; unnecessary, 46, 49–51, 59–60, 63, 65, 69, 75, 81, 94
bisphosphonates, 27, 29, 62
Black, William, 92
bladder cancer, 48
blame, necessity of, in U.S. legal culture, 163
blindness, 15, 17
blood clots, 32, 41–42, 44, 62, 165, 168
blood donation, 211n10
blood pressure: defined, 2–3; low, dangers of, 12–13, 27. *See also* hypertension
blood sugar, dangers of low, 16, 19, 27
Bloom, David, 41
body mass index (BMI), x
Boston, 32–33
Bozeman, Montana, 180
brain cancer, 176–77
brain hemorrhage, 2, 92
Brain Tumor Foundation, 176, 178
Brawley, Otis, 156
breast cancer, 29, 61, 62, 73–88; Betty Ford effect, 84–85; BRCA1 and BRCA2 genes for, 122, 127, 212n19; deaths, 77, 85, 148–49; diagnoses, 77, 85–87, 206n20; ductal carcinoma in situ (DCIS), 86; effect of regular screening on the amount of cancers detected, 87; incidence, 84; overdiagnosis of, 75, 77, 82–84, 86–88, 119; preventive mastectomy for, 119; reservoir of, 206n18; risk, 132, 148–49, 205n9; screening for, 73–75, 78, 81, 83–86, 143, 204n8; spectrum of abnormality of, 77–78; surgery for, 73, 79, 87–88. *See also* mammography
Breast Cancer Action, 77
Bretz, J. Harlan, 181–82, 189
Bristol-Myers Squibb, 24
Britain. *See* United Kingdom

British National Health Service, 150
bulging disks in back, 44; study of asymptomatic people, 36
Bush (George W.) administration, 76

Canada, 182
Canadian National Breast Cancer Study, 75, 82, 86, 89
cancer: changing genome in, 134; dangers of treatment, 45, 52; fast-growing, 53–54, 78, 80, 162, 164, 183; genetic risk of, 117–18; Gleason score, 130; heterogeneity of progression, 53–54; metastasizing, 61, 79, 162; nonprogressive, 54, 97; overdiagnosis of, 45, 53–54, 60–61, 71–72, 89, 96, 100, 134, 165–67; overtreatment of, 45, 70–71, 88, 99, 130–31, 134; paradigm shift in thought about, 53; pathologic definition of, 145; phobia, 165–66; problem of genetic variability in, 133; as a pseudodisease, 54; screening, xii, 45, 53, 60, 72, 89, 98–99, 137; shift in biology of, 53; slow-growing, 53–55, 97; spectrum of abnormality in, 50; of the vocal cords, 90. *See also* incidentalomas; *individual types of cancer*
candesartan, 28
Cardiac Arrhythmia Suppression Trial (CAST), 103–4
carotid arteries, 43; recommendations against screening, 113; stenosis, 113
Catalona, William, 51
Centers for Disease Control, 89
cervical cancer: overdiagnosis of pre-cancerous abnormalities in, 69; Pap smear for, 70, 194n1; screening, 70; treatments, 70
cervix (in pregnancy), 188–89
cesarean section (C-section): because of overdiagnosis, 105–6, 110; complications of emergency, 105; increase in, 105–6, 209n4
chemotherapy, 73, 88, 134

chest pain, 1–2

cholesterol: argument for testing children's, 28; borderline, 99; changing definition of, 20–21; defined, 15; distribution by level, 22; and financial alliances of people entrusted to define, 24, 155; high, 15; high-density (HDL), 21; and increase in treatment from changing definition, 21, 155; low-density (LDL), 20–21; overdiagnosis of, 25–26; overtreatment of, 21; and risk of heart disease, 21, 127; screening of children, 28

chronic pelvic pain syndrome, 166

Cleveland Clinic, 48

clinical exam compared to diagnostic technology, 41–42, 74–75, 86

clubfoot, 111–12, 168–69

Cochrane Collaboration, 105, 112

Cochrane's Review, 88

cognitive impairment, xi, 12, 186

Collins, Francis, 118

colon cancer: familial adenomatous polyposis gene for, 127; fecal occult-blood test for, 147; overdiagnosis of precancerous abnormalities, 69; removal of polyps, 71; screening for, 71, 147, 162

colonoscopy, 101, 165

Colorado, 43

colposcopy, 70

Columbia River, 182

Columbia University Medical Center, 113

condition: chronic, xiii; defined, xvi

Congress, 182

Connecticut River, 31

Copernicus, 118

C-section. See cesarean section

CT scans, xi, 32, 38, 63, 95, 147; anxiety from, 93, 97; chest, 35, 91–92, 164; in diagnosing abdominal aortic aneurysm, 39, 41; kidney, 96, 98; number of, 35; in overdiagnosis, 34, 44, 92, 97, 119, 166; sinus, 34; whole body, 38, 95, 101. See also spiral CT scan

cystic fibrosis, 121, 123–24, 134, 210–11n4

cysts, kidney, xi

cytology, 67

Dartmouth, NH, 151

Dartmouth-Hitchcock Medical Center, 113

Dartmouth Medical School, xvi

deCODEme (company), 116

dehydration, 12

dementia, xiii

Denmark, 83

Department of Health and Human Services, xiii, 76, 182

Department of Veterans Affairs (VA), 1, 10, 21, 151–52; hypertension study, 3–4, 5–6, 12

depression, 11

dermatologists, 30, 65–66

diabetes: A1c test in, 196n4; borderline, 99; changing definition of, 18; coma caused by, 17; defined, 15, 17–18; effects of, 15, 17; effects of intensive therapy on, 19, 196n4; and financial alliances of people entrusted to define, 24, 155; glucose tolerance test for, 189; and increase of treatment from change in definition, 18, 155; mild, 18, 168–69; overdiagnosis of, 16–17, 27, 168–69; risk factors, 126, 189; and risk of heart disease, 127, 196n4; spectrum of abnormality in, 17–18; type 1, 17; type 2, 16–17

diagnosis, x; anxiety from, 47, 119, 165–66, 169, 171, 188–90; epidemic of, xii, 140, 156, 174–75; excessive, xiv, 30–31, 60, 160; increasing, xii, xiv, 174–75; patient demand for, 175; prior to symptoms, danger of overdiagnosis, 15, 45, 119, 155, 184–85; of risk of a disease, 116–19; as a self-reinforcing cycle, 174–78, 180; spectrum of abnormality in, 172–73; surprise, xiv, 34, 139, 157, 164. See also early diagnosis; harm

diagnostic technology, 42

diagnostic tests, xi, 93, 100, 160, 175;

increase in, 160, 167; and intolerance
of uncertainty, 164–66; and overdiagnosis, 166

diarrhea, 60

disease: advocacy groups, 136, 157–58, 160,
186–87; awareness campaigns, xi, 159;
defined, xvi

DNA, 116, 120, 123, 134, 135; junk, 127–28;
producing different phenotypes in
different environments, 134. *See also*
genetic variants

Doll, Sir Richard, 68–69

double helix, 116

Down syndrome, 108–9

ear, nose, and throat doctor, 90, 139, 142

early diagnosis: bad outcomes following,
141, 143, 163; better health care by,
xiv, 102, 167; both sides of the story,
148–50, 168–69; dilemma of, 178–79;
exaggeration of benefits, 136–38, 141,
148, 150, 186–87; favorable outcomes
following, 140–41, 143, 173; fear,
use of in promoting, 137–38, 160;
financial interests in, 157–60, 167;
as a goal, xv; hurricane analogy for,
178–79; increasing medical costs, 157;
increasing survival without prolonging
life, 144–45, 149, 187; lead-time bias
in, 144–46, 212n5; marketing of, 137;
misuse of survival statistics, 137–38,
140; need of a randomized trial for,
147–50, 186; need for skepticism
regarding, 183–85; overdiagnosis
from, 137–38, 143, 145–46, 150, 184–
85; overdiagnosis bias in, 145–47;
paradigm of, 182, 184; patient demand
for, 151; personal anecdotes about, 137–
41, 150; point of negative return from,
184; potential benefits of, 170–71; to
prevent bad events, 15; problems with,
60; questioning the value of, 86, 98–99,
180, 183–84; true belief in, 15, 102, 151,
157–60, 167, 180, 182; value of, 135, 162

electrocardiogram (EKG), 2; defined, 102–3

Emanuel, Kerry, 179

emphysema, 67, 99

endocrinologist, 30, 62

endoscopy, 30, 160

enthusiasm: for early diagnosis, xii, 110,
115; for genetic research, 127, 133; for
medical technology, xii; for scanning,
101–102; for screening, 37, 101–2, 113,
174–76, 187–88

epidemiologist, 156

epileptic seizure, 91

esophagitis, 30, 62, 169

Europe, 83, 84

evolutionary biology, 116

Expert Committee on the Classification of
Diabetes Mellitis, 17–18

extrapolation, excessive, 173–75

eye hemorrhage, 6

falls. *See* hip fracture

FDA. *See* U.S. Food and Drug
Administration

fear: of malpractice, as a factor in overdiagnosis, 164; used in promoting
screening, 137–38, 160, 175–78, 186–87

fetal monitoring: effect of, 106; evidence
of benefit from, 105; and increase in
C-section rates, 105–6; overdiagnosis
from, 106–7

Filly, Roy, 107–9

financial interests: in disease awareness
campaigns, 159; "doing well by doing
good," 158; ethical argument over, 156;
against a free market in medical care,
154–56, 214n5; of increasing the market
for treatments, 24, 28, 65, 153, 155–56,
185; in overdiagnosis, 151, 156–58, 180;
as a reason to not treat, 10; in setting
numeric rules, 15, 24; in vascular
screening, 113

finasteride, 119

Finland, 63

Ford, Betty, 84–85

Forteo, 152–53

Fox Chase Cancer Center, 139

Fracture Intervention Trial, 26
Framingham Heart Study, 37, 198n6
free-market system, 154

gallstones, study of asymptomatic people, 36, 44
gastroesophageal reflux, x
gene: mutation, 123; therapy, 116
genetic: aberration, 123, 211n8; abnormalities, 134; counseling, 109, 112; diseases, 116; research, 117, 123, 127, 129, 133; risk as one factor contributing to disease, 132
genetic disease: cystic fibrosis, 121, 123–24, 134; hemochromatosis, 123–25; Huntington's disease, 121–23, 134
genetics, 116, 118; effect of environmental factors on, 120; explained, 120; is not destiny, 120; over 99 percent is identical in all people, 120; spectrum of disease-gene penetrance, 122–23
genetic selection and preimplantation genetic diagnosis, 212n19
genetic testing: arguments against, 124–26; defined, 116–17, 120–21; false sense of immunity from, 132; overdiagnosis in, 116–19, 123, 126–27, 130, 133–34; to predict future phenotypes, 121; profit motive, 116; unintended side effects of, 119
genetic variants, 123, 132, 211n8; BRCA1 and BRCA2, 122, 127, 134; C282Y, 124–27; effect on phenotypes, 128; familial adenomatous polyposis, 127; and prostate cancer, 128–29; single nucleotide polymorphisms (snips), 127–29; weakly penetrant, 123
genome scan, 117–19, 133, 168
genotype, 121, 124–26; associated with liking Brussels sprouts, 121; defined, 120
Geologic Society of America, 181
Georgetown University Medical Center, 113
Georgia Cancer Center at Emory, 156
Gerstein, Hertzel C., 19
Glacial Lake Missoula, 181–82

GlaxoSmithKline, 24
glucose-6-phosphate dehydrogenase deficiency, 116
glyburide, 16–17
Google Earth, 38
grant money, 158
Great Salt Lake, 39
Gulf of Mexico, 179
gynecology, 107

harm: from diagnosis, 170, 172–74; economic, from overdiagnosis, 10, 164, 170; emotional, from overdiagnosis, 31, 37, 51, 165, 168–69; emotional, from overtreatment, 47; physical, from overdiagnosis, 20–21, 25, 30, 51, 60, 74, 146, 165, 168–69; physical, from overtreatment, xv, 12–13, 19, 45, 58, 99, 168–75
*Harrison's Principles of Internal Medicine*, 20
hassle factor as a reason to not treat, 10, 169–70
health, pursuit of, 185–86, 190–91
health-care reform: "death panels," 76; obstacles to, 180; politics of, 76–77, 89, 143, 215n9
health-care-reform law of 2010, 66
health-care system, xiii; increasing costs of, 180; introduction of disease and disability by, xiii
health insurance, 35, 119, 170; denial of, 66, 126, 143, 170
Health Insurance Plan of Greater New York (HIP): breast cancer study, 74–75
Healthy People 2010, xiii
Healy, Bernadine, 76
heart attack, 2, 184; prevention, 13, 15, 27, 103; risk factors, 21, 29; and risk of heart disease, 21
heart disease, 17, 40; risk, 21, 117–18, 126–27, 132
heart failure, 6
heart transplantation, 102
Heath, Iona, 88

hematologist, 165

hemochromatosis, hereditary, 123–26;
  bloodletting as treatment for, 124,
  126, 211n10; diagnostic approach, 125;
  harm from overdiagnosis of, 126; iron
  overload from, 126; overdiagnosis of,
  125; penetrance, 126

heparin, 165

hepatic cell adenoma, 93

high blood pressure. *See* hypertension

High Uintas, 39

Hill, Sir Bradford, 68–69

hip fractures, 152–53; prevention of, 153, 160;
  as risk factor for death, 13, 153

hoarseness, 90–91, 168

Hopper, Dennis, xii

hormone replacement therapy (HRT), 5;
  and risk of other diseases, 29, 61–62,
  85, 132, 194n7

Human Genome Project, 118

Huntington's disease, 121–23, 134

Hurricane of 1938, 179

hydralazine, 4

hydrochlorothiazide, 4, 12

hypertension: borderline, 99; changing
  definitions of, 2, 20, 27–28, 155, 196n4;
  crisis, 3; diastolic, 5, 8, 12; effects
  of, 3; essential to deliver blood to
  organs, 3; and financial alliances of
  people entrusted to define, 24, 155;
  mild, x, 8–9, 12, 168–69; moderate,
  8–9; overdiagnosis of, 1, 20, 27; and
  risk of aneurysm, 40; and risk of
  heart disease, 21, 127; severe, 2–3, 5,
  8–9, 13–14, 168–69, 185; spectrum
  of abnormality in, 13; studies, 5–8;
  systolic, 11–12; treatment, 3, 5, 12–13,
  194–95n6

hypothyroid, 142

Illinois, 181

imaging technology changing the rules,
  32–33, 44

impaired healing, 17

impotence. *See* sexual dysfunction

incidentalomas, 90–101, 208n14; anxiety
  from, 96, 98; defined, 91–92;
  epidemic of, 97; incidence, 92, 94–95;
  overdiagnosis of, 94–95

incontinence, 60

infection, 17, 184

infotainment, 160

insulin, 17

International Osteoporosis Foundation, 24

intervention: early, 102; from genetic
  testing, 118, 132–34; preventative, 11,
  173; skepticism about, 11, 13, 174. *See
  also* treatment

Italy, 83

Jarvik artificial heart, 102

Joint National Committee on High Blood
  Pressure, 20, 27

*Journal of Ultrasound in Medicine,* 107

Kaiser Permanente of Northern California,
  104–5

Katete, Zambia, 33

kidney cancer, 91, 95–98, 100; overdiagnosis
  of, 96–97, 168–69

kidney failure, 6

Lake Michigan, 181

laryngitis, 90

Lauer, Matt, 51

lawyers, 143; as a driving force in overdiagnosis, 98, 151, 161–63; jokes, 161.
  *See also* liability concerns

Legs for Life (company), 113

leukemia, 62–63

Leukemia and Lymphoma Society, 139

liability concerns, 65, 100, 161–63, 180. *See
  also* lawyers

life: expectancy, xiii; insurance, 3. *See also*
  quality of life

Lifeline (company), 113

liver cancer, 93–95

living longer, yet sicker, xii–xiii

London, 68

lung cancer, 47, 61, 69, 99, 185; dangers

of surgery, 67–69; deaths, 66, 68; diagnoses, 66, 95; overdiagnosis of, 67; risk identification, 67, 90, 95; screening for, 182; spiral CT diagnosis of, 68–69

macular degeneration, 117–18
malaria, 116
mammography: anxiety from, 81–82, 88, 119; because of genetic risk, 119; benefits of, 74–82, 87; both sides of the story, 148–50, 213–14n12; diagnostic, 73, 82, 88; financial interests in, 159; harm from, 75–76, 79, 81–82, 87, 119; and health-care costs, 76; lead-time bias in, 144–45; overdiagnosis from, 145–46, 205–6n16; politics of, 76–77, 89, 161; proportion of cancers detected by, 205–6n16; required insurance coverage of, 182; screening, 73–76, 78–79, 83, 85, 143, 148–49; by socioeconomic status, 144; and spectrum of risk, 78; standardization, 89
Massachusetts General Hospital, 32–33
Mayo Clinic, 41
Mayo Lung Study, 67
media role in overdiagnosis, 180, 186–88
mediastinum, 91
medical care: best in the world, xii; better by early diagnosis, xiv; expansion of, xii, xvi; paternalistic model of, 155; problems with profit motive in, 154; quality of, judged, 154–55
medical-industrial complex, 156
Medicare, 35, 65, 67, 107
medication adherence, 3
melanoma (skin cancer), 61, 64–66
Mendel, Gregor, 116
meniscal damage, 36, 198n6
Merck, 24
metabolic acidosis, 17
Miami, 179
Minnesota, 39
miscarriage, 108–9
Montana, western, 182
Montana State University, 180–81

MRI, 32, 35, 37, 92, 176, 198n6; in overdiagnosis, 36, 44, 91, 93, 137
Mulroney, Brian, 69

Napoli, Mary-Ann, 156
National Breast Cancer Coalition, 77
National Cancer Institute (NCI), 63, 74, 75, 76, 85, 156; "50,000 tumors, 40,000 aberrations," 133; PDQ (Physician Data Query), 89
National Heart, Blood, and Lung Institute, 19
National Institutes of Health, 19, 75, 76
National Osteoporosis Foundation, 23, 28
National Women's Health Network, 77
Navigenics, 116
NBC (network), 41, 51
New England, 137, 151, 179
*New England Journal of Medicine,* 37, 128
New Mexico, 80
*New York Times,* 60, 76, 110
New Zealand, 159
nodules, 46, 91, 99–100; lung, xi, 69, 92, 95; thyroid, 62
Nolan, Brian, 115
North Lake Mall, 156
Norway, 83, 86
Novartis, 24
numeric rules: for cholesterol, 20–21; concern about the experts who set, 24; for diabetes, 17–18; effect of changing and adding of millions of patients, 16, 18, 21, 23–24, 27–28, 32; financial interests in, 15; for hypertension, 2–3, 8, 11–12, 27; importance of, 15; for osteoporosis, 23; in overdiagnosis, 16, 24–25, 50–51; for prostate cancer, 50–51

Obama, Barack, 143; administration, 76
obsessive-compulsive disorder, xi
obstetrician, 107, 111, 188–89
oncologist, 46, 156
Oregon, 33
osteopenia, 30, 168–69

osteoporosis: and algorithm to determine risk of hip fracture, 29; changing definition of, 23–24, 28, 155, 197n24; dangers of overtreatment for, 27, 61–62; defined, 15, 22–24; early diagnosis of, 22; effects of, 15; and financial alliances of people entrusted to define, 24, 155, 160; medication for, 152; overdiagnosis of, 26–27, 30. *See also* T score

osteosarcoma, 153

ovarian cancer: BRCA1 and BRCA2 genes for, 127; screening, 182; surgery because of genetic risk, 132, 212n17

overdiagnosis: defined, xiv–xv, 25. *See also* harm

overtreatment, xv, 28–31, 119, 150, 165, 185. *See also specific conditions*

pancreatic cancer, 185

pancreatitis, 69, 92

paradigm shift, xv, 1, 3–4, 13, 18, 53, 180; difficulty in effecting, 181–82

Pardee, Joseph, 181

pathologists, 63, 83

patients, drive to turn people into: by doctors, 1, 32, 46, 82, 155; by drug manufacturers, 24, 156–58; by government, 27–28; by the medical establishment, xvi–xvii, 18, 21–22, 31, 113–14, 180

pediatrics, 33

"perfect market" for medical services, 154–55

peripheral artery disease, 113

pertussis vaccine, 4

PET scan, 32

Pfizer, 24

pharmaceutical companies: financial interest in overdiagnosis for, 151, 153, 155–59; marketing by, 46, 152, 157–59; representatives, 151–53

phenotype, 125–26, 134; defined, 120; trumps genotype, 121, 123, 128

phlebotomy, 124

physical exam compared to diagnostic technology, 39–41, 89. *See also* clinical exam compared to diagnostic technology

Pittsburgh, 68

placebo, 4, 28, 103–4, 195n8

pleurisy, 164

pneumonia, 67, 96, 99, 165, 184

polyps, 33–34

potassium, 17

prediabetes, 28

pregnancy, 104–10, 188–89, 209n7. *See also* amniocentesis; sonogram

prehypertension, 27, 197n9

premature birth, 104–5, 188–89

preosteoporosis, 30

Prevention Health Screenings, 113

Priceline.com, 153

prostate: benign hyperplasia, x; benign hypertrophy (BPH), 10, 57; biopsy, studies of, 49–50, 200n6

prostate cancer, 45–61; biopsy for, 46–47, 49–52, 58, 60–61; genetic variants associated with, 128–29; new deaths from, 56; new diagnoses of, 56, 58; overdiagnosis of, 45, 49, 51–52, 55–59, 119, 130, 168–69, 202n22; preventive prostatectomy, 119, 131; reservoir of, 48–49, 57, 130, 200n4; screening for, 58, 60, 131, 147, 164, 168; surgery, 47, 56–58; transurethral resection (TURP), 56–58

prostate-specific antigen (PSA), xi, 50–52, 58, 174; change in threshold for biopsy, 51, 60, 119, 201n10

prostatitis, 166

Provo, Utah, 39

PSA. *See* prostate-specific antigen (PSA)

PSA test, 162, 187; and argument over what is an abnormal level, 46, 50–51; because of genetic risk, 119; "The Great Prostate Mistake," 60, 168–69; overdiagnosis from, 57, 59, 130; "profit–driven public health disaster," 60

pulmonary embolism, 41–42

pursuit of: disease, 185, 190; health, 185–86, 190–91

quality of life, 190–91; defined, xiii; improvements in, 174

radiation, 32, 58, 73, 88; risks of, 74, 93
radioactive iodine therapy (RAI), 139, 142
radiologist, 33, 80, 88, 91–93, 96, 98–99, 107, 160, 164–66
randomized trial: for abdominal aortic aneurysm screening, 147–48; for arrhythmia, 103–4; for breast cancer, 73; for cancer screening, 137; for cholesterol, 21–22; for colon cancer, 147; defined, 4–5, 194n6; for diabetes, 19; for hormone replacement therapy, 29–30; for hypertension, 5–9, 12–13, 27–28, 194–95n6; for lung cancer, 67, 147; of mammography, 74–75, 86, 88, 147–49, 205n10; for osteoporosis, 26–27, 152; for premature birth, 104–5; price of, 136; for prostate cancer, 201n17; for PSA testing, 59, 147; treatment groups in, 5–9, 13, 27–28, 103–4, 194–95n6; on value of early detection, 147–48
Raynaud's disease, x
Reagan, Ronald, 69
rectum, 58, 187
reserpine, 4
risk: absolute, 130–32, 148–50; defined, 131; identification, xii; lifetime, 25, 26, 130–32, 205n9; measured over years, 5–8, 13, 28–29, 58, 114–15; relative, 131, 148–49, 213n7
RNA, 116
Road to Early Detection (brain scanner), 176–77
Rochester, Minnesota, 41
Rocky Mountains, 180
Roosevelt, Franklin D., 3
Royal College of General Practitioners, 88

San Francisco, 32
scanning. See screening
Schwartz, Lisa, xvii, 52, 107–8, 177, 188–90

Scopes monkey trial, 118
screening, xiv, 38, 47, 157, 176–77; campaigns, 176, 186; does not reduce mortality, 99; enthusiasm for, 174–76, 188–89; and false positive results, 75, 81–82, 110, 149–50, 176–77; financial interests in, 136; as a loss leader for hospitals, 156; as a manner to be considered competent, 161; overdiagnosis in, 34–35, 99, 178, 187, 190; paradigm of, 102; as the path of least resistance, 161, 189–90; positive-feedback loop in, 177–78, 187, 215n3
Sebelius, Kathleen, 76
SEER. See Surveillance Epidemiology and End Results program (SEER)
Senate Appropriations Committee on Labor, Health, Human Services, and Related Agencies, 76
sexual dysfunction, 47, 51, 58, 60, 169
Shatner, William, 153
Should I Be Tested for Cancer? (Welch), xiii
sickle cell disease, 116
sigmoidoscopy, 162
sinusitis, 45, 91; overdiagnosis of, 33–35, 44
skin cancer, 48
smoking: and risk of heart disease, 21, 127; and risk of lung cancer, 67–69, 92; and risk of osteoporosis, 29
snips. See genetic variants
sonogram, 105–13; abnormalities, 108–12; added cost to pregnancy from, 109; added miscarriages from, 108–9; anxiety from, 107–8, 110–12; "The Best Way to Terrify a Pregnant Woman," 107–8; dangers of, 108; no benefit from, 112; overdiagnosis from, 108–10. See also ultrasound
Specter, Arlen, 76
spectrum of abnormality, 78; in abdominal aortal aneurysm, 40; in cancer, 50; in diabetes, 17–19; in hypertension, 9–10, 13; and potential benefit and harms from diagnosis and treatment, 171–72, 215n1; in treatment, 172–73

spinal compression fracture, 174; defined, 152

spiral CT scan, 42, 68; overdiagnosis from, 68–69

statins, 27

steroids, 29

streptomycin, 4

stroke, 13, 29, 37, 43, 44, 186, 195n7; silent, 37–38

Surveillance Epidemiology and End Results program (SEER), 56, 63, 79, 80, 84, 97, 201n13

Sweden, 83

symptoms: as an indicator of effective intervention, 184, 216–17n5; as one of the best predictors of serious problems, 183

tamoxifen, 87, 119

tendonitis, 36

testing: anxiety over, 119, 177–78, 191; as a measure of medical quality, 161; as the path of least resistance, 161

thrombosis, deep venous, 41

thyroid cancer, 30–31, 61–63, 95, 138–40; new deaths from, 62, 64; new diagnoses of, 62–64; overdiagnosis of, 63, 138, 140, 168–69; papillary, 63; reservoir of, 63, 203n3; side effects of treatment, 142–43; surgery, 64, 139

thyroid gland, 30, 203n1; biopsy, 30, 62–63, 139, 142; nodules, 62; synthetic hormone, 139, 142

*Today Show,* 51

transient ischemic attack, 43

treatment, 5, 15–16, 25, 33–34; because of overdiagnosis, xv, 24, 27, 44, 58, 119, 180; better health from, xiv; cancers resistant to, 162, 164; downside of, 13–14, 139; increase in, xiv, 31, 42; selling to the well, 151–53; spectrum of abnormality in, 172–73; unnecessary, xv, 29–31, 35, 61, 93, 147–48, 180. *See also* benefit of treatment; *specific conditions*

trisomy syndromes, 108–10, 210n10

troponin level, 2

true belief in early diagnosis. *See* early diagnosis

T score, 15, 22–23, 29–30

tuberculosis, 4, 194n1

23andMe (company), 116

ulcerative colitis, 16

ultrasound, 32, 39, 41, 43, 46, 189; overuse of, 40, 44, 62, 63. *See also* sonogram

United Kingdom, 4, 38–39, 83–84, 149–50

University of Arizona, 60

University of California at San Francisco Medical Center, 32, 107–8

University of Maryland Medical Center, 113

University of Pennsylvania Medical Center, 113

University of Utah Medical Center, 102–3

University of Washington School of Public Health, 85

urologist, 71, 96, 98, 162

U.S. Food and Drug Administration, 153

U.S. Geological Survey, 181

*U.S. News & World Report,* 33

U.S. Preventative Services Task Force, 58, 63, 76, 77, 106–7, 112–13, 125, 182

U.S. Public Health Service, 33, 102

Utah, 39

VA. *See* Department of Veterans Affairs (VA)

vascular screening, 113–14

ventilation-perfusion scanning, 42

Vermont, 10–11

viruses, 116, 164

Warm Springs Reservation, 33, 34

Wasach Range, 39

Washington (DC), 176–77

Washington (state), 181

*Washington Post,* xii–xiii, 178

Welch, H. Gilbert: career, 32–33, 102, 151–52, 177, 180–81; education, 85, 154; health, x–xi; published works, xiii

White River Junction, VT, 1
White River Junction VA hospital, 90
Whitmore, Willet, 71
whooping cough, 4
Woloshin, Steven, xvii, 52, 96, 177, 189
World Health Organization, 23, 24, 29
World War II, xii–xiii

X-rays, 32, 152; abnormal, xi; in bone
    mineral density testing, 22, 197n11;

chest, 68, 99; in overdiagnosis, 33–34,
    67, 90–91, 95–96, 164–65

Yellowstone ecosystem, 180–81

Zambia, 32